Praise for
Refuse to Regain!

"Losing weight is incredibly difficult, and keeping it off is even harder. In *Refuse to Regain!*, Dr. Berkeley combines equal parts science, experience as a practicing physician, and common sense to offer a no-nonsense prescription for success."

—Mitchell A. Lazar, M.D., Ph.D.; Director, Institute for Diabetes, Obesity, and Metabolism, University of Pennsylvania

"Do you honestly want to keep off the weight you've lost? You will find this ground-breaking book your best friend and guide to accomplish that goal. Based on a wealth of experience, sound reasoning, a keen understanding of human nature (as it functions in our modern food-rich environment), and a firm grasp of the best in nutritional science, Dr. Barbara Berkeley has developed an intelligent and effective formula."

—Anthony Sebastian, M.D.; Professor of Medicine, University of California San Francisco

"After 25 years of books about losing weight, there is finally a resource to guide patients and the dietitians who work with them during weight maintenance. This book gives nutritionists the tools to help clients fully understand what lifestyle changes need to be made to ensure success. A must-read for health care professionals working in weight management."

—Darlene Paluf, RDLD

"Dr. Berkeley has done a superb job of presenting a practical, easy to follow lifetime plan for eating that is virtually consistent with the diet to which humans are genetically adapted. This book is lively, to the point, and transforms difficult scientific concepts into easily understood explanations."

—Loren Cordain, author of *The Paleo Diet*, *The Paleo Diet for Athletes*, and *The Dietary Cure for Acne*

Refuse to Regain!

Refuse to Regain!

12 Tough Rules to Maintain the Body You've Earned!

by Barbara Berkeley, M.D.

Quill
Driver
Books

Fresno, California

Printed in the United States of America.

Published by
Quill Driver Books
An imprint of Linden Publishing
2006 S. Mary, Fresno, CA 93721
559-233-6633 / 800-345-4447
QuillDriverBooks.com

Quill Driver Books may be purchased for educational, fund-raising, business or promotional use. Please contact Special Markets, Quill Driver Books, at the above address or phone numbers.

Quill Driver Books Project Cadre:
Doris Hall, Linda Kay Hardie, Christine Hernandez,
Stephen Blake Mettee, Kent Sorsky, Cassandra Williams

First Printing

ISBN 978-1884956-93-5 • 1-884956-93-9

To order a copy of this book, please call
1-800-345-4447.

Library of Congress Cataloging-in-Publication Data

Berkeley, Barbara, 1948-
  Refuse to regain! : 12 tough rules to maintain the body you've earned!
/ by Barbara Berkeley.
     p. cm.
  Includes bibliographical references and index.
  ISBN-13: 978-1-884956-93-5 (hardcover)
  ISBN-10: 1-884956-93-9 (hardcover)
  1. Weight loss. I. Title.
  RM222.2.B4527 2008
  613.2'5--dc22

                                                            2008029704

For my daughters,
Ariel and Kayla

Contents

The production staff moved quickly and quietly, guiding me to my mark behind the closed stage door. Dressed in skinny black jeans, a tight off-the-shoulder knit shirt, a wide-studded belt and suede knee boots, I looked nothing like the woman in the photo montage playing for the audience on the other side. For a moment I felt like I was her again—sadness filled me as I watched my photos on the monitor fade one into another as my voice told the story of how I got to be nearly 300 pounds.

I looked away and took a deep breath. This was no time for self-doubt. I was meeting Oprah in a few seconds and the producers expected me to walk out on stage with attitude and confidence.

I exhaled. "Come on out!" said Oprah, and the stage door sprung up. The audience gasped—and then cheered. The energy of their applause propelled me on to the stage and I left behind the insecure woman in the monitor. With a broad smile and hips swaying, I walked over to weight-loss expert Bob Greene and gave him a hug; then Oprah embraced me and said privately, "You look great."

I was one of twenty-one people on the show that day who had lost a significant amount of weight through diet and exercise. Standing on stage with everyone at the end of the show, I looked around at their happy faces and it dawned on me that, as wonderful as this was, losing the weight was merely the ship revving up its engine, and being on Oprah was no more than the bon voyage party for the real journey ahead: maintenance.

I reached my weight-loss goal on a cloudy March day in 2007. I was at my doctor's office for a routine checkup. I weighed 138 pounds. I said to my doctor, "So, do you suppose I'm done?" She said, "I think you can stop now." And that boring little exchange was how I became what Dr. Berkeley calls a POW—Previous Overweight Person. There was no fanfare, no confetti, no fireworks, no angels flying around the room singing "Hallelujah." Just me, my doctor, and my medical file, in which my doctor wrote, "Lost 158 pounds in two years, two months and twelve days."

I walked out of her office no longer a person losing weight, but a person maintaining my weight. I got in my car, sat there for a moment, and thought, "Now what?"

I'd been on countless diets in the past and the few times I reached my goal I celebrated with food, essentially saying, "Finally! I can go back to the way things used to be." But this time was different. I was different. I didn't want to celebrate with a Dairy Queen Oreo Blizzard and a corn dog. I wanted to figure out what to do next so I wouldn't go back to the way I used to be, regaining weight. I wanted off that merry-go-round.

I went to the book store and found it woefully lacking in texts pertaining to weight maintenance. One could get lost in the shelves of diet books and still spend fruitless hours searching for a comprehensive plan on what to do when the "dieting" is over.

I researched the Internet and found bits and pieces of information about maintenance, mostly mixed in with the larger topic of weight loss. I increased my food intake by a few hundred calories a day and yet in the ensuing weeks was still losing weight. I worried to the point of obsession about every food choice, each minute of exercise. Was it enough? Too much? Was it normal to still lose weight even though I was eating more?

During this time, my weight-loss story and blog were featured on a CNN FitNation segment. I received an email from Dr. Barbara Berkeley, who found my story interesting, particularly the fact that I'd kept an online journal throughout my weight loss. She was searching for ways to support weight maintainers and asked if we might work together on an Internet support site. To get the discussion started, she sent me a copy of Refuse to Regain! 12 Tough Rules to Maintain the Body You've Earned! From the first chapter, I knew this book was the maintenance tool I had longed to find months before.

The Refuse to Regain message is strong and clear: maintenance requires diligence and planning. It requires adopting a warrior mentality to navigate the real world of modern food consumption and to say no to would-be saboteurs. It requires understanding the body's

Foreword

response to complex and simple sugars, fat, and protein; developing and sustaining an exercise regimen; and nurturing our emotional health by seeking out others in maintenance for support. These pages contain concrete guidance to help those who have lost weight and are determined to keep it off.

As a writer needs a pen and a carpenter needs a hammer, POWs need a fundamental, basic tool to help them navigate the treacherous waters of weight maintenance. We need reliable, no-nonsense information. Refuse to Regain shines a light in the dark void left empty by a world obsessed with weight loss and ignorant to the true challenge that is weight maintenance.

Whether you've lost 10 pounds or 200, *Refuse to Regain!* is an indispensable companion on your journey toward permanent weight control.

Lynn Haraldson-Bering

Acknowledgments

Publishing a first book is a daunting task. I want to sincerely thank all of those who helped along the way and believed in the value of this project.

Special thanks to my Oliva Schwartz for helping this book move from just a thought to pages on paper. Her advice, enthusiasm, and encouragement were vital to this process. To my literary agent Linda Konner, many thanks for taking on a difficult project and making it work. Thanks also to Dr. Julie Silver and the staff of Harvard Medical School's nonfiction publishing course for giving me the opportunity to present my work to those who could best move it forward. I am also grateful to Kathy Dawson, who was unselfish in her willingness to share what she had learned as a published author and who got me on the right road.

Thanks also to Frank Greicius, M.D.; Kate Mills; Linda Koenig; Beverly Glick; Faye Wenger; Denny Linden; Marge Zebrowski; Loren Cordain, Ph.D.; Mitch Lazar, M.D.; Anthony Sebastian, M.D.; and my website partner, Lynn Haraldson-Bering for their help and contributions. A special thanks to Chef Matthew Anderson for his tireless (and good-natured) work on creating and reworking recipes to conform to my "Primarian" requirements.

To my terrific partner Darlene Paluf R.D.L.D and my talented staff: Kim, Carlene, Peggy, Kelly, Mira, and Julie, thank you for your hard work every day and for being so tolerant of the endless talk about this project. I'd also like to express my thanks to all those patients and friends who read and reviewed parts of this book. To all of my patients at Weight Management Partners, thank you for sharing your struggles, your triumphs and your wisdom.

Unending gratitude to my parents, Frieda and Jerry, and to my sister Hope, for providing the love that is the rock of my life. Thanks to my daughter Kayla for her superb technical support and to my daughter Ariel for making health and wellness her career.

Refuse to Regain!

And, as always, to my amazing husband Don, who continues to believe in me and not only tolerates my crazy dreams, but makes them come to life.

I doubt you'd think of me as the typical doctor. Often, when I see my patients I'm wearing sweatpants, sneakers, or tennis clothes. Most of my clients don't mind. They are old friends by now. I know about their families, their jobs, their car troubles, even their pets. That's because they are all engaged in the long process of controlling weight, and my staff and I are right there in the battle with them.

For a good part of my career, my specialty has been the medical management of obesity. It's all I do, and sometimes—to hear my husband tell it—all I think about. While most doctors would prefer to leave weight management to someone else, I'm fascinated by it. Since 1988, when I first became involved in the field, I've been working with, reading about, and observing people just like you. I've seen you lose weight and, unfortunately, I've often seen you regain every pound.

Regain is a depressing, seemingly inevitable frustration for most dieters and we professionals haven't done much to help you out. I want to change all that.

The road to wisdom is not always obvious. My academic training includes a master's degree from Columbia University, a medical degree from the State University of New York, and a residency in internal medicine at a Harvard teaching hospital. I've been the medical director of a large hospital-based obesity program and, for the past eight years, director of my own weight management practice.

Credentials are nice. But the most valuable information I've learned about weight management has come not from academic pursuits but from my patients. Experience with real people takes on particular importance when you work in a field that is plagued by contradictory research studies, questionable food pyramids, and a large number of "experts" who don't actually treat overweight patients.

Perhaps you are frustrated, as I am, by daily headlines that proclaim a particular food healthy one day and poisonous the next. You may be utterly tired of trying to figure out how many grams of this, that or the other thing will save you from nutritional doom. Often, these diet pronouncements come from research studies. But doing good nutritional research is very difficult. Many studies come to conclusions based on what subjects remember having eaten. Those participating may be asked to write down how much and what types of food they consumed over long periods. Often, their memory is faulty. As a result, the conclusions that are drawn can be faulty too.

So what we learn from experience is important. And this is a book based on my experience working with weight maintenance patients. Some of the recommendations inside may be unfamiliar to you. I urge you to give them a chance as they represent techniques that work in the real world.

Perhaps it will help if I add that, in addition to being a weight loss doctor, I am also a weight maintainer. For the past five years, I have successfully kept off twenty pounds by spending each day using the techniques I recommend in this book. So, I can give you the benefit of both a personal and a professional perspective. Let me assure you that following this plan is both very possible and very effective.

Finally, remember that your experience qualifies you as an expert too. So be sure to read this book and all diet information critically. See if the recommendations make sense given what you know about yourself and your weight issues. Consult your own instincts as you proceed. Adopt those things that resonate and discard those that don't. The goal is to find a plan that works for you.

Together, I hope we can make your current weight loss your final one.

Barbara Berkeley, M.D.

Altered Foods: Foods of the past 100 years which are changed, added to or otherwise manipulated.

Diet of Conviction: A named diet which represents someone's strong beliefs about food.

Food Assault: Unwanted intrusions of food into a maintainer's life.

Food Creep: The tendency for more food, particularly S food, to creep back into your life.

Gong Food: An intensely flavored S food that simulates a ringing bell when consumed.

Life Charter: A well-considered plan for eating and health that is your personal guideline for living.

Maintenance Junior: Derived from "Just Reduced," a person who is just beginning the process of maintaining weight.

Modern Foods: See Newcomer Foods

Newcomer Foods: Foods introduced with the advent of agriculture, about 10,000 years ago.

NOW: Never overweight.

Plate Pattern: The automatic division of your dinner plate into areas of Primarian eating.

POW: Previously overweight.

Primarian: Someone who eats a diet exclusively composed of primary foods.

Primary Foods: Foods that come mostly unchanged from nature and could have been eaten by ancient man.

Revenge Clothes: The form-fitting clothes that look great on you now that you're thinner.

Scan and Plan: A technique for visualizing each day's eating challenges.

Scream Weight: A weight set by the maintainer that he or she never wants to exceed.

Second Hand Food: Like second hand smoke. The presence of unwanted food in a confined area.

S Foods: Foods that turn into sugar in the bloodstream. Sugars and starches.

SLIM: Someone who is at the Senior Level in Maintenance. A person who is maintaining their weight skillfully.

Thrill Eating: The sport of eating just for the fun of it.

Weight Mentor: A senior maintainer who has reached the highest level of skill and commitment.

Weight Permanence: Maintaining goal weight without deviating.

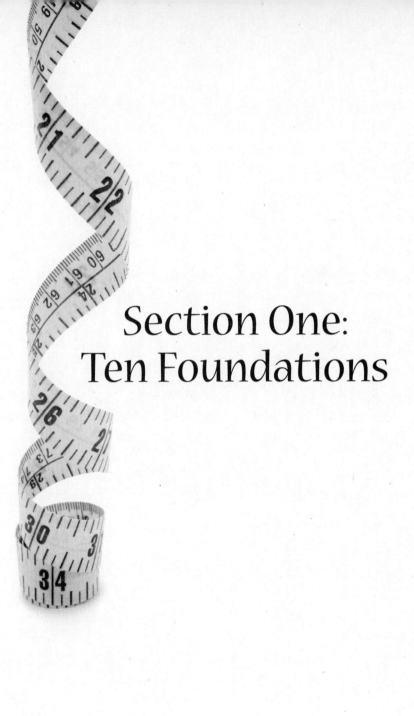

Section One:
Ten Foundations

Chapter One

The Maintenance Junior

If you would know the road ahead, ask someone who has traveled it.
—Chinese saying

Even though we've not yet met, I can tell you that I admire you. I have two good reasons for feeling this way.

The first is my respect for your successful weight loss. Whether you reached your goal through diet, prodigious amounts of exercise, medications or surgery, there are simply no easy ways to lose weight. Your weight loss means that you were able to set a tough goal and see it through—a true accomplishment. A recent poll from the Harvard School of Public Health surveyed a sample of overweight people and found that over half of them were trying to diet at any given time. That's a lot of calorie counting. Yet you didn't just diet; you succeeded in getting the weight off.

But you have another quality that impresses me even more. You have the ability to see and face facts. At a time when many people might be binging and celebrating, my guess is that you identify more with the following:

> "Most people who lose weight gain their weight back. In fact, I've regained before. How can I prevent that from happening again?"

That's smart thinking. And you're right to be concerned. For many who've lost weight, a big celebratory moment marks the end of dieting. After all, the diet is over, isn't it? This is exactly the miscalculation that starts the lose and regain cycle.

You, on the other hand, are approaching things differently. You're feeling appropriately uncertain about your remodeled body with its new needs and challenges and about your own ability to make your permanent changes. These feelings, while disconcerting, show that you have good instincts. Continue to follow them!

Refuse to Regain!

I can tell you from experience that *all* successful dieters are determined to stay at their new weight and never to return to old eating patterns. But they fail with depressing regularity. Want a simple proof? Write down the names of everyone you know who has ever lost weight. OK, forget writing them down; that chore could take a while. Instead, list all of those whose pounds have stayed off. Did your pencil even touch the page? Many research studies have confirmed the fact that keeping off lost weight is rare.

But does any of this say anything about you? It doesn't have to. I believe that dieters regain not because they are trapped in some inevitable cycle, but rather because of an unfortunate lack of guidance. Through no fault of their own, people who lose weight go into the next phase— the maintenance phase—without a single strategy. Failure soon follows.

Let's put an end to that situation right now. Maintaining lost weight is a lifelong journey. You can have a wonderfully successful outcome if you acquire a strong knowledge base and follow a good roadmap. You can also benefit from traveling with a guide who knows the often-rugged terrain. Fortunately, these elements and supports are exactly what appear in the pages that follow.

With your permission, I'll help you. I'll prepare you, outfit you, and point out potential pitfalls as we go. I can do this because I've traveled this road before. Who am I? I'm a physician—an internist—who stumbled into the weight-management field by accident, fell unexpectedly in love with it and made it my career.

In 1988, when I had two young daughters to raise, I was offered a hospital-based job running a large weight management program. This opportunity seemed like a good way to avoid the middle-of-the-night calls most physicians live with and mark time until my girls were old enough for school. Like most doctors, I had little interest in trying to convince people to lose weight. Normally that's a very difficult task and believe it or not, just twenty years ago, obesity was not the pressing problem it is today. We knew much less then about obesity's connection to the diseases that plague modern society nor did we foresee the enormous weight epidemic that was to come. Although I was less than enthusiastic about my new assignment, it seemed a good way to combine M.D. and M.O.M., so I took the job.

To my utter surprise, I soon found that helping people with weight loss was thrilling. The reason? When our patients lost fat they became healthy in so many other ways. Their high blood pressure, diabetes, cholesterol problems, arthritis, acid reflux disease, irritable bowel, sleep apnea and other problems either improved markedly or disappeared. In addition, their struggles with weight were fascinating and touching.

Inspired by them, I started to pay more attention to the pressures that society and advertising exerted on eating habits. I learned about ways in which foods were engineered to make them more irresistible. I began to see patterns in food consumption that reminded me of the patterns of people with addictive drug problems. Suddenly it appeared as if modern foods and our modern way of consuming them were at the center of absolutely everything: emotion, addiction, compulsion, and most of all—disease. I was hooked.

Since the 1980s an entire science of obesity has developed, complete with its own societies and journals. I formed my own private obesity practice and have continued to treat, read, and observe. While much of what we have learned about fat and how it behaves is quite new, one thing has not changed: the most important thing we can do is help those who have lost their excess pounds stabilize their weight. This permanent effort is called weight maintenance.

When you lose weight, you become what I call a POW, someone who has been "Previously Over Weight." You may look like a NOW (a "Never Over Weight" person), but the resemblance is an illusion. In fact, your bodies and metabolic processes are quite different.

Suddenly it appeared as if modern foods and our modern way of consuming them were at the center of absolutely everything: emotion, addiction, compulsion, and most of all—disease.

Everything you've achieved weight-wise means nothing if you can't maintain. Isn't it strange, then, that so little is written about how to achieve permanence? POWs are a vastly underserved group. This book is my attempt to fill that void for you.

What Is a Maintenance Junior?

At this stage, you are what I call a Maintenance Junior, and please believe me when I say that I know you well. I've heard your stories, seen your triumphs and bemoaned your failures. What I believe most about you is that no matter what the statistics say, you can succeed in staying right where you are: at a good weight and in much improved health.

Maintenance Junior is the term I've come up with to describe those who, like you, have Just Reduced (that's the source of the "J.R." or "junior"). I also like the term Junior because it expresses the idea of inexperience. Maintenance Juniors tend to be babies in the big, bad food woods. It is likely they are in need of practical guidance, education, and support. What a shame that Maintenance Juniors often leave weight-loss treatment at the very moment they need help most. Juniors have conquered the weight barrier and feel they can conquer the world. "Now that I've lost weight, keeping it off won't present a problem," they think. Big mistake. *The skills required to maintain weight differ markedly from those required to lose it* and Maintenance Juniors do not yet have these skills. While Juniors are powerfully convinced that they will never return to old ways, they almost always do.

Acclimating to Maintenance Junior status is a bit uncomfortable, I know. It means dealing with the feeling of going from the top rung of experience to the bottom. Just yesterday you were someone who defeated the scale, an expert dieter. Today, you find yourself facing the challenge of lifelong dietary change, a very real shift in scenery. It will help greatly if you can accept the fact that you will be a maintenance rookie for a while and vulnerable to mistakes of inexperience. These may include:

- Feeling overconfident
- Trying to go it alone
- Underestimating the challenge ahead
- Believing there is no need for additional knowledge
- Having a weak plan or no plan at all
- Relying on moderation

Time to Look Squarely at the Challenge

Of all the errors to which Maintenance Juniors are prone, the most dangerous is underestimating the task they face. As I said, maintenance is a journey and the terrain can be rugged. Like any other adventure, though, the challenge can be exhilarating. Allow me to direct your attention upward and let's look unblinkingly at the mountain you've set out to climb.

Just how hard do you think it is to maintain weight? While no one has exact figures about how many maintainers achieve permanence, all agree that the vast majority do not. In 2000, the University of Michigan tracked the weights of 854 community members for three years. Only 4.6 percent lost weight and kept it off and that was during a very brief period of maintenance. In another report published in the *Archives of Internal Medicine*, a group of 192 successful dieters were studied, each of whom had an average weight loss of about forty-five pounds. After three years, almost 90 percent of the group had gained back most or all of the weight. Worse, 40 percent of the dieters weighed more than they had when they started. These kinds of results are typical of published reports about long-term weight control.

The figure you hear bandied about is that 95 percent of those who lose weight soon regain. But let's be generous and make the assumption that as many as 20 percent of those who lose weight keep it off permanently. Given this, we have a basis for comparing the difficulty of weight maintenance with the difficulty of completing other tasks. In terms of degree of challenge, how does maintenance stack up?

Task	Percent Who Successfully Complete Task
Getting through marine boot camp	85%
Finishing law school once accepted	90%
Marathon starters who finish the race	82%
Getting into medical school (all applicants)	37%
Completing college once accepted	55%
Successfully buying a home (U.S. citizens)	70%
Successfully getting to the top of Mt. Everest	20%
Maintaining a significant weight loss	20%

A bit sobering, isn't it? The failure rate for maintenance (80 percent or greater) approximates the failure rate for one of the most difficult challenges in the world—climbing Mt. Everest! Remember, though, that this failure rate reflects the attempts of all sorts of people, most of whom have not had any specific guidance in the skills of maintenance. Clearly, to complete any of the tasks on the list above, a person needs intense preparation, planning, motivation, and the willingness to persevere. For each of these tasks, there are plenty of people to help. Somehow, despite the fact that avoiding regain is one of the toughest jobs on the list, similar supports are not available to maintainers. We need to arm you with the same set of skills that would get you a house, a medical degree, or through a marathon finish line. And that's the point of this book.

Mount Everest Versus Mount Maintenance

The forces that oppose challengers to Everest and challengers to weight regain are formidable. Mt. Everest throws the power of nature against the climber at every turn. Similarly, the Maintenance Junior is faced with a blizzarding food culture, burying him or her with seductive messages, stimulating the appetite, and subverting attempts to succeed. We will learn more about this in chapters to come.

As I said earlier, preparation is key. How does someone get ready to climb Mt. Everest? He or she might prepare for years getting in top physical condition, securing the latest equipment, and selecting the best guide. Each possible route would be studied and the experiences of past climbers carefully dissected. Only when all was in place would the climber set out for the mountain, prepared as thoroughly as possible to undertake one of the world's greatest challenges.

How about the average Maintenance Junior? How does that person prepare for a challenge that creates as many failures as Everest? Unlike our climber, he or she doesn't have the luxury of years to prepare, nor a ready source of equipment, guidance or route. In many cases, the Maintenance Junior hasn't even been eating a normal diet, and is fresh from a regimen of bacon rinds or liquid supplements. With few successful role models to consult, there is no one with whom to discuss strategy. Worst of all, the mountain in the distance doesn't look so big from the new maintainer's perspective. It seems to be a small hill, easily climbed with a few tweaks to daily habits. Maybe I can give you a realistic idea of Junior expectations by reproducing some actual conversations from my office practice.

These are responses given by Juniors when asked: "Now that you have completed your weight loss, what is your plan for maintaining your new size permanently?"

- "I am going to eat healthy because I have to change my lifestyle."
- "I know I really have to exercise more."
- "I have to stay away from junk food."
- "I'm going to do what my thin friends do: they eat in moderation."
- "I'm going to limit my portions and try not to eat desserts."
- "I have a whole gym in my basement."
- "I'll only eat the bad stuff once in a great while."

At first blush, these might seem to be reasonable answers except when we look at them in light of the extreme difficulty of weight maintenance. None of these responses tells me that the speaker has a specific, detailed plan. Without a plan and the determination to carry it out, there is bound to be failure.

Let's imagine we are asking a group who is about to climb Mt. Everest how they plan to do it and we get the following answers:

- "I walked up some hills at home to prepare."
- "I don't have a guide, but I've got some maps."
- "I'll stay away from the edge of the mountain."
- "I'll climb during the week but not on the weekends."
- "I'll get there by being moderate in my approach."

I don't think any of these climbers should proceed past base camp, do you?

It's all about the specifics. The tougher the challenge, the more detailed the plan must be. But you don't like plans, you say? Sure you do. Your recent weight loss is the best example of a plan that worked. Your effort was successful because you accepted the premise that it was impossible to lose weight without following a strict regimen. It is immaterial whether that plan was eliminating all carbohydrates or drinking pots of cabbage soup. Your dedication to a routine and your persistence in getting it done was the key to your getting to goal.

People say that they don't like the idea of permanent regimentation, but in fact all of us spend our lives following ongoing plans. We never think to reset them. We go to work each day rather than just when we feel like it. We tell our kids to brush their teeth every day, not when the spirit moves them. We study for school and attend classes consistently, not just a day or two a week. In fact, most of our lives consist of repetition. Routines that accomplish vital business are not optional. Having an eating and fitness plan is a routine that accomplishes something of prime importance. *We abandon it at our peril.* Believe it or not, it is just as possible to condition yourself to a permanent weight loss plan as to brushing your teeth each day. But consistency and tenacity are key.

Your personal Everest will not include snow, gale winds, or dangerous drops, but it will feature formidable obstacles. You will need equipment and strategies to avoid each one. I hope to provide them. Let's look at the challenges you will face on your particular mountain.

Challenges of Mount Maintenance

1. **The food avalanche:** You live in a food flood, an entire culture devoted to encouraging you to eat. Expect to be buried and make sure you have the tools to dig out.

2. **Habit crevasses:** You have eaten in a certain way for a lifetime and have come to expect food to serve particular functions. It is easy to fall into a rut you can't get out of. For many Maintenance Juniors, a major relearning process is needed to break habits such as comfort eating and what I call "thrill eating."

3. **An icy metabolism:** You have just lost weight, but the fat cells that contained that weight are still a part of your body. Biochemical signals that accompany weight loss may prompt you to eat, and will need to be overcome. In addition, your genetic tendency to gain weight easily still remains. Although you may look slim, you are actually a POW (previously overweight). You do not have the physiology of a never-heavy person, something you will need to respect.

4. **Climber's fatigue:** Losing weight was an exciting, attention-getting makeover. Permanence requires a relentless, daily attention to detail that no one but you may notice. This phase will only work if you learn to deeply love the new you and the very process that allows you to stay as you are. Not only can you do this, but it will also be highly rewarding.

5. **Bad trail markers:** There is a lot that can lead you in the wrong direction in commonly accepted nutritional wisdom. This is particularly true in regard to foods that are appropriate for the POW. Many of the foods that we consider staples are easily eliminated without harmful effect; in fact, their elimination is key for POWs.

6. **Inadequate conditioning:** Climbing any mountain, whether real or figurative, requires physical strength. As the years pass, it is almost impossible to achieve permanence unless you establish an athletic identity. We will discuss this more as we go on.

7. **Dangerous footing:** Travel, stress, occasions both happy and sad, all provide opportunities for slippage.

8. **Sabotage:** The very friends and family who love you may have trouble with your healthful habits and may try to overturn your efforts at permanence. It's not personal. It just is.

Now that we've looked at our mountain, let's lay out the ropes and lines we'll use to get to the top. Here are the methods we'll employ:

Coaching

Your first step is to believe you can succeed. Throughout this book, my job will be to provide you with truthful information about the challenges of maintaining weight and about the processes that will help you do it. Sometimes my message will be tough. I will ask you to accept uncomfortable facts and to make big changes, not moderate ones. I will do this for a single reason: I want you to become permanently healthy. Remember that most coaches create winners by asking for performance. When it comes to tough tasks (like avoiding regain), it is commitment and seriousness of purpose that works. This approach is what I will ask you to bring to our work together.

Techniques

My goal in this book is to give you simple, practical guidance for changing the way you look at eating and at food over your lifetime. My test for each guideline consists of asking the following questions:

- Is this behavior easy to understand?
- Is it easy to put into practice?
- Is it effective?

The only way to get permanent success is for the way you live to become second nature. Counting every calorie, tallying up fat percentages and the like are not behaviors that fit easily into a busy day. The 12 Tough Rules which make up Section Two are simple, effective and will form the structure of your life in maintenance. Following these rules will assure your success. Learning to enjoy them will change your life.

Facts

I have always been impressed that despite all of the detailed nutritional information that consumes pages and pages of most diet books, very few of my patients know much about basic food science. Perhaps this is because we're too hung up on what *The New York Times* recently described as "nutritionism." That is our fixation with the components of foods: cholesterol, folic acid, omega fats, and so on. We have become so involved in the complex micro-contents of our diet that we've forgotten what food is. For this reason, I have tried to simplify science and stick to the basics. In the first section of this book, I have laid out the information that will help you most. I ask you to read these chapters carefully because they form the foundation for the behaviors I will ask you to practice. Learning more is always encouraged, but is optional.

Insights

Together we will look at what has worked for other people who have avoided regaining weight. This information is available both through data collected in studies and by speaking directly to those who are keeping weight regain at bay every day. In the third section of this book, we will talk to five people who are maintaining weight in the real world. We won't dwell on their achievements. What we want to know is: what works for them and how can you put the same skills into practice.

A tough message

It's hard to say if anyone really believes that pounds can "Melt Away," that you can "Think Yourself Thin," or that you can drop weight on the "Pizza Lover's Diet." Yet these are the messages that magazine covers continually deliver about weight. Diet books are slightly better, but most of them still shrink from telling the whole truth. What good is pretending that controlling weight in our food-crazy world is easy? I can't imagine any benefit to that pretense and I won't add to it. Years of experience with patients have taught me that maintainers like you want honesty. Throughout this book, I will ask you to do some hard work to maintain this new body of yours. I said this was a journey, so get your boots on and welcome the challenges with a resilient spirit.

How Do We Know that Weight Permanence Is Possible?

Having read this introduction you may be thinking: "This is pretty daunting. Is weight permanence really achievable?" The answer is, very definitely! We actually know more about successful maintainers than ever before thanks to a landmark study called the National Weight Control Registry. This study, begun in 1993, currently includes about 6,000 people, each of whom has lost a minimum of thirty pounds and has kept the weight off for at least a year. (If you have lost this much weight,

I hope you will soon join this study yourself). Current participants are doing quite a bit better than even these numbers suggest. On average, they are maintaining a loss of about sixty-five pounds and have kept that weight off for five and a half years. To make this all the more impressive, these are not people who have found weight loss easy in the past. About 70 percent of the participants were overweight during childhood or teen years, a characteristic that is usually associated with stubborn obesity in adulthood. Almost everyone in the study group (90 percent) tried unsuccessfully to lose weight before finally getting it right. Clearly, something changed these previously frustrated regainers into effective long-term maintainers. Perhaps the best news of all, however, is that once two to five years have passed, the chances of achieving *permanent* success appear to become much greater.

So get comfortable with your status as a rookie, a Maintenance Junior, for the next year or so. Think of it this way: you can achieve your goals by taking a very real look at the challenges ahead and by learning how others have negotiated the same obstacles. You're unlikely to master this information if you dismiss maintenance as simply "not doing what I did before." Spend some time on the bottom rung and before you know it, you will be a Senior Level Maintainer helping someone else climb the ladder.

Chapter Wrap

- A Maintenance Junior is someone who has recently lost weight and now seeks to stay at his or her new size.
- Maintaining weight takes skills that are quite different from the skills learned during dieting.
- Juniors tend to be overconfident about their ability to keep weight from returning.
- Following a plan and having a guide for maintenance is crucial.
- Approaching the task ahead with a tough attitude is vital.

Chapter Two

Become a Warrior:
Banish Guilt and Commit Yourself

When it becomes necessary to do a thing, the whole heart and soul should go into the measure, or not attempt it.
                        —Thomas Paine, *The Rights of Man*

It is one thing to talk about committing yourself to a task, but quite another to do it. In this chapter, I'd like to talk to you about the importance of serious commitment to your maintenance efforts and about an issue that often prevents Maintenance Juniors from getting to their goal: guilt.

Making a commitment means making a promise to follow through, both to yourself and to others. The word commitment is used to describe our relationship to especially important vows. We are committed to our life partners, our religious values, and our work. Why is it so important to view your year as a Maintenance Junior with the same intensity? First of all, your body is your base of operations. All of your other commitments rely on how well you take care of it. The determination to stay healthy, then, assumes prime importance. Second, and very simply, you will relapse unless you decide to make a real commitment to maintenance.

We all cast around for explanations as to why we fail to maintain the weight we've lost. Could it be something about our metabolism? Something lacking in the way our bodies are built? We don't have to look that far. In reality, dieters gain weight back for the most obvious of reasons: they fall off the wagon.

Recently, an interesting article in the *American Journal of Clinical Nutrition* supported this. Researchers noticed that the weight loss of obese people on diets was often small, much less than what would be expected given their size and diet plan. Was their small loss due to a metabolic problem or to something else? To find out, the researchers studied three potential explanations.

It was possible, they reasoned, that obese people absorbed more of what they ate than other people. If they did, they might "squeeze" more calories out of each portion than normal weight people would and thus lose less than expected when dieting.

A second theory suggested that the metabolism of obese people might drop to very low levels during dieting. A super sluggish metabolism might prevent dieters from losing weight no matter how few calories they were given.

...your body is your base of operations. All of your other commitments rely on how well you take care of it.

The third theory was the most obvious one. This proposed that subjects failed to lose weight because they did not stick to their food plan well enough. To figure out which theory was correct, researchers reviewed all available studies on each topic. The result?

- No study showed that overweight people absorbed food differently than thin people.
- No study suggested that overweight people who dieted had abnormal changes in metabolism.
- The authors concluded that the problem was failure to fully adhere to the prescribed diet.

A second study of low-calorie dieters supported this conclusion. Participants were treated in a weight loss program, followed for one year, and asked to rate how well they stuck to their diet. Levels of "sticking to it" started to fall off immediately after the diet began and continued to worsen throughout the year. The few study participants who did manage to follow the diet completely lost appropriately large amounts of weight, as opposed to the smaller losses of others.

If we debunk the theory that diet failures are due to imperfect metabolism (more of this in Chapter Eight), we are left feeling guilty for a failure of willpower. Nearly every dieter has felt this destructive emotion as he or she struggles with the daily battle with weight.

Guilt plays a large role in motivating our eating behaviors. We start dieting because we feel guilty about allowing ourselves to get too fat. We beat ourselves up with guilt throughout the diet process when we have bad days. We are overwhelmed with guilt when we can't keep off the weight we've lost. This guilt-fest leads me to ask two vital questions:

1. Are dieters completely to blame for what they perceive as their lack of willpower?
2. If not, who or what else might be responsible?

It's Not Your Fault

If you can identify food-guilt in yourself, I'd like you to work on getting rid of it. Guilt disables you and prevents you from keeping your eye on the goal. Guilt makes you feel weakened and ashamed. I hope to convince you that guilt has no place in maintenance.

Yes, it's true we often can't stick to our eating plans. It's true we regain weight. But we rarely go beyond our own guilt to ask why this is. Time to take a good look. Are you the only one responsible for the difficulty you experience in keeping your commitment? Or are other forces contributing to your guilt and failures? I believe that, in truth, you have nothing to feel guilty about. You are simply being outmaneuvered.

Societal views contribute to making us feel ever more responsible for our own lack of control. Food producers and sellers are comfortable with the idea that overeating is a personal failing. After all, no one is forcing you to eat the stuff they make and market to excess. In order to keep selling food, they would like you to believe that you are just someone who makes poor choices. Unfortunately, many other voices perpetuate this belief.

Contributions to your guilt come from everywhere. A couple of years ago I attended a citywide conference on obesity. A federal official spoke on the skyrocketing weights of children. After the speech, I asked the speaker if the government would consider banning TV food ads that targeted children. This is not a particularly radical idea. Pulling ads for health reasons has precedent. The hard liquor industry, for example, enforced a self-imposed ad ban after Prohibition (recently lifted), and in 1971 the government stepped in to remove cigarette ads from the airwaves. Wouldn't it make sense to prevent the marketing of unhealthy foods to our most vulnerable citizens—kids? The federal official saw things differently. In his view, a child's food choices were entirely up to the parent, a matter of the family's personal responsibility. In other words, parents of overweight kids were guilty of harming their children, but those who inundated their children with thousands of craftily constructed food ads were not. Do you believe this to be true? I don't.

Are we and our children overweight simply because we make irresponsible choices? With overweight and obesity levels approaching 70 percent in the U.S., this would lead us to conclude that the vast majority of our population is lacking in willpower. Yet the supposedly irresponsible citizens who allow their families to get too fat are the same people who own successful businesses, raise productive children, buy and maintain their own homes and earn advanced degrees. No. Americans are not short on willpower, nor do they lack personal responsibility. I believe that they are simply overwhelmed by what Yale psychologist Kelly Brownell calls a "toxic food environment." They also suffer from lack of useful education on proper nutrition, a subject that remains sadly ignored in schools and in the training of health professionals.

It is easy for food makers, restaurants, naturally thin people, and even your own government to lay the blame for obesity at your door. You are the wimp, the weakling, the one with no willpower, they claim. No wonder you are riddled with guilt. Well, don't fall for it.

You are having trouble controlling food because marketing and the continual availability and nearness of food are controlling you. How so? We all know that the human mind is malleable. It is easily influenced. Here's an example: have you ever seen someone under hypnosis? Within a few moments, the hypnotist is able to take a relaxed and receptive mind and use it to plant a suggestion. Suddenly, a businessman in a three-piece suit is walking like a chicken! Despite this demonstration of the power of suggestion, most of us remain certain that we are immune to influence and are completely able to think for ourselves.

To put this idea to rest once and for all, we need look no further than the American advertising industry. This business, worth multibillions, would not exist if each one of us were not influenced by pictures, slogans, jingles, and messages. A 30-second commercial in the 2007 Super Bowl cost as much as $2.7 million, cash that would never be spent unless marketing had the proven power to change our behavior. In 1999, the amount of money spent on convincing you to eat food was $7.3 billion. Just to break that figure down, that included $765 million on candy and gum, $549 million on soft drinks, and $330 million on snacks. You begin to see the magnitude of influence that invites Americans to eat, eat, eat. And believe me, you are susceptible to this onslaught.

It is possible to avoid manipulation, but only if you maintain continual awareness of attempts to sway your thinking. It helps to keep your eyes and ears open, to be completely clear on your position, and to associate with like-minded people. Even so, when it comes to eating and food, you are up against not only powerful food marketers, but also an entire culture, which is happily and mindlessly eating. That's a mighty dose of persuasion.

Now that we've established the power of the forces enticing you to eat, imagine this scenario: someone puts little you in a boxing ring with a giant 10,000 times your size and weight. The giant takes one swing and knocks you out in five seconds. You wake up on the canvas. As you return to consciousness, what's in your mind?

Are you feeling guilty? I don't think so. You might have two black eyes and a mighty headache, but I don't think you'd feel guilty about your defeat. What might you be feeling instead? You might feel completely hopeless and decide that you couldn't possibly win a rematch. You might, therefore, give up. Or, you might be angry at being subjected to such an unfair fight. Your determination to win might lead you to think of some diabolic tricks that would allow a lightweight like you to beat up a big brute.

Each day, millions of us arise from our beds feeling guilty about having been knocked out by a food giant. When you feel the temptation to beat yourself up about your lack of willpower, remember that you are up against enormous commercial and cultural pressures in your battle to lose and maintain weight. You are not weak, lacking in spirit, or without willpower. Instead, I encourage you to think of yourself as a noble warrior in a very tough fight, one that is truly worth winning. Periods of failure and backsliding are normal—but guilt is simply not appropriate. Quitting the fight is always an option, but it is one I hope you will avoid. If you choose to stay in the ring, use every crafty trick in the book to outwit your enormous opponent. The first is to eliminate the burden of guilt from the forces that are already weighing you down.

You Are a Warrior

Being a warrior is serious business. Let's explore the concept further. The Random House Dictionary offers this definition: a person who shows great vigor, courage or aggressiveness. We generally think of a warrior as someone who:

- Is prepared for combat.
- Has a clear sense of the enemy.
- Belongs to a group of other fighters.
- Has a sense of mission in his or her quest.

Unless you're Don Quixote, it's hard to war against something harmless. Try working up a righteous anger against disco music or reality TV, for example. Our western culture makes it hard to get mad about obesity by treating it as a trivial problem, not something worth getting upset about. On the one hand, we bemoan our overweight state. On the other hand, we are not particularly alarmed by our heaviness. We even find it funny. Overindulging and getting fat are generally accepted as minor human foibles, not as serious threats to our national health. In the next chapter you will learn that just the opposite is true. In fact, fat has deadly consequences which cause our health to suffer not just when we become obese, but as soon as we begin to gain excess weight. I ask that you read this scientific information carefully. It will help provide the motivation that keeps you going during maintenance.

A Warrior's Commitment to Health

Most diets apologize for themselves by telling you that you'll soon be able to add back the foods you love or that simply making small changes to current behaviors will be enough to make long lasting change. I want you to come at things from an entirely different perspective. I want you to welcome significant change as a way to opt out of our unhealthy food environment. I ask you to do this by first making a commitment to true health.

When you were losing your weight, did you ever say, "I'm doing this for me"? People often do. When I ask patients what that means, they say that they want to be healthy. But they usually don't realize that "doing this for me" can have two meanings. When you are doing something you perceive as good for yourself long-term, like saving for retirement or pumping iron, you feel virtuous. But doing things that make you feel good immediately is also a form of "doing something for me"... a more pure, pleasurable and self-indulgent form. Examples are: eating cake and candy, drinking alcohol, buying things on impulse, and watching TV when you should be cleaning the garage. Without making any value judgments, which of the following activities gives you a feeling of "doing for me" more?

1. Reading the classic novel you've always wanted to conquer or following the exploits of Brad and Angelina in People Magazine?
2. Running five miles on the treadmill or lounging on a beach chair with a mystery novel?
3. Buying a very safe car with airbags placed every two inches or buying a gorgeous convertible?
4. Eating a plateful of salad and broccoli or having a Death by Chocolate Brownie Delight?

While each of these activities is something you do for yourself, one involves realizing long-range goals and the other indulging immediate desires. Both of these types of activities have a place in your life, but it's important to see how easily one type of "doing this for me" can overrule the other.

Focusing on the tasks that lead to long-term reward requires a mind adjustment. To accomplish these tasks, you must override a tendency toward adolescent thinking. We live in a world of immediate gratification and that world is reflected in the way we eat. We're able to indulge our immediate wants by having endless goods and services at our fingertips. Want lobster for dinner? It's on the next corner. A new DVD player? Choose from twenty-five models at your local computer store. How about a new nose? You can have one tomorrow. Long-range planning and forgoing the pleasures of the moment for future reward are adult behaviors. Impulsive, live-for-the-moment decisions are consistent with the behavior style of adolescents. Perhaps you believe as I do that our world of highly available gratification encourages us to act more like teenagers than like the grown-ups we really are.

Simply put, it's much easier to give in to the plate of nachos in front of us than to imagine its consequences in some far-off future.

I encourage you to think of yourself as a noble warrior in a very tough fight, one that is truly worth winning. Periods of failure and backsliding are normal—but guilt is simply not appropriate.

Successful weight maintenance requires you to spend a good deal of time in adult mode, considering scenarios that are many years ahead. What will you be like in ten years if you regain? In twenty? Can you create a picture of two futures: one in which you are eighty years old and running a senior marathon, and a second in which you are in a nursing home with diabetes and a hip replacement? This takes adult thinking. The information you will read in the chapters ahead is about you and your potential future. As a warrior in the weight maintenance arena, I ask you to step forward and take responsibility for it.

Tactics: Offense/Defense

New Zealand's Maori warriors developed a fascinating tradition for pumping themselves up before battle. They performed a ritual dance and chant called "haka" which included shouting, grunting, making fierce faces, pumping fists, and jumping up and down. The haka is still performed today by a number of sports teams, most notably the "All Blacks," one of New Zealand's rugby teams. If you have never seen a haka, you can easily do so by searching the term on YouTube. While I don't advocate your jumping out of bed each morning and bellowing like John Belushi in Animal House, I do think that the haka teaches us something about staying on the offense.

Since maintaining weight is a conflict, you will always want to stay on the offensive side of the ball. If food is beginning to rule you, the balance of power has changed and you are simply trying to ward off disaster...you're on defense. You can increase your opportunities to be on the offense by following a routine (as you'll learn), and also by creating you own motivators. Create some on your own or try these:

1. Keep a picture of yourself on your refrigerator door at your original weight and one at your current weight. Some people prefer to hang other motivational pictures, such as photographs of people who inspire them.
2. Keep a favorite pair of pants or piece of clothing that fits you snugly hung on the outside of your closet. Put it on each day before getting dressed.
3. Wear a meaningful wristband or pin each day. One possibility: the Lance Armstrong "LiveStrong" yellow band (available from the Lance Armstrong Foundation at livestrong.org). Like a string tied around your finger, these pieces remind you of your daily goal.
4. Review every day in your mind before you set out. Anticipate the food challenges and prepare an action in response.
5. Develop your own mini-haka, a chant or mantra that gets you going.

Chapter Wrap

- The process of maintaining weight is a battle between your resolve and the world which is constantly encouraging you to eat.
- In taking on this battle, you are doing something very meaningful. Be proud.
- Expect challenges.
- Get rid of guilt.
- Act like a warrior.
- Remember the real long-term reasons you are in this battle. Stay on the offense by planning and executing.

Chapter Three

When Fat Is Fatal:
Metabolic Syndrome and Other Nasties

Weight sits like a spider at the center of an intricate, tangled web of health and disease.

—Walter Willett, M.D., *Eat, Drink and Be Healthy*

If you read only one chapter in this book, please read this one. It holds the key to your motivation for permanent weight control. If you are to make deep-seated and long lasting changes in your life, there must be a reason to do so. What is that reason for you?

Is it because you look and feel better? These are certainly important reasons for wanting to stay slim, but they tend to fade over time. In several months, it may become hard to remember how you felt before your weight loss. As time goes on, friends and family (and even you) will get accustomed to your new size. When this happens, many of the positive reinforcements you associated with losing weight will be gone. Lacking these motivators, you may well be tempted to seek out other things that make you feel good. These may include ice cream, chips, and brownies. Throughout your life in maintenance it will help to remember that there is a much more compelling reason to fight the fight than your jean size. The reason is simply this: regaining your weight has the very real potential to kill or disable you. People who are effective maintainers have a healthy respect for the lethal side of fat.

Lethal? Most of us don't think of fat as dangerous. At best, it's a cuddly layer of jiggle—at worst, a frustrating annoyance. But life-threatening? For many years we doctors believed, like you, that fatty areas were undesirable but harmless. We thought that the body's millions of fat cells were simply fuel tanks full of energy, uncomplicated and unthreatening. We were seriously mistaken. The past few years have opened our eyes to the fact that fat tissue can be extremely nasty stuff.

Forgive me, but I'm going to attempt to scare you. I want you to be fully aware of the fact that approximately 300,000 people died last year because of medical problems caused by being too fat. I want to shake you up enough for you to become deadly serious about your determination to refuse to regain.

Perhaps you are about to skip this chapter because you are one of those people who tolerated being overweight with perfect blood pressure and without a single abnormal blood test. If you think that this gives you a free pass, please read on. Research recently reported by Northwestern University studied over 17,000 people of varying size who had neither cardiac disease nor diabetes at the outset. Many appeared, like you, to be at very low risk for developing future medical problems. These low-risk people had normal blood pressure, normal cholesterol and were non-smokers. They were then followed for several decades. What happened? Over time, those who were overweight—even those whose blood tests were initially normal—had a higher risk of hospitalization for diabetes and heart disease and a higher risk for death than did normal weight people. Those who had normal blood tests but were obese turned out to have four times the risk of developing heart disease and eleven times the risk of dying of diabetes than did normal weight people.

What does this mean for you? It means that you don't want to gain your weight back even if everything tested "normal" when you were overweight. Lots of extra pounds just aren't good for you. Complicated lab tests aside, remember that your heart is about as big as your fist. It is simply not intended to power an overlarge body. Over time, this mismatch takes an inevitable toll.

Perhaps you're a maintainer who was never that heavy to begin with. Surely, if you gained back that ten or twenty pounds, it wouldn't be much of a threat to your health? I suggest you to read on, too. Data from the Harvard Nurses' Health Study shows that your chances of developing diabetes, high blood pressure, heart disease, and gallbladder disease begin to rise markedly not when you become obese, but as soon as you start to gain even small amounts of weight.

It should be a no-brainer. Keep the weight off. You're about to learn more about why this is by far the smartest course.

How Can Fat Hurt You? Let Me Count the Ways

Fat can harm you in mechanical ways and in metabolic ways. The distinction is important. The mechanical load that extra weight puts on the body is obvious. Clearly, knees were not built to lug around fifty unexpected pounds. Ditto hips, ankles, and feet. Other mechanical problems occur when the weight of a large chest, belly, and throat disrupt breathing at night (sleep apnea) or when a big abdomen pushes acid out of the stomach during sleep (gastric reflux). These problems, while disabling, are unlikely to threaten your life. But there is a hidden and deadly side of fat that can.

Fat tissue takes on a new and dangerous profile when it settles around the middle of the body, an all too familiar location for most of us. The fat you can grab with your hands is not the problem. But this external belly is a marker for fat inside the abdominal cavity. This internal fat, called "visceral" fat (meaning around the viscera or organs) is not the quiet little storage depot we thought it to be. Instead, it is a highly active endocrine tissue. This means it makes things. In fact, visceral fat is a busy factory pumping out some pretty nasty chemicals and hormones.

Let's take a direct look at this belly fat. The picture below is the CAT scan of someone who is overweight. Since you're not a radiologist, allow me to orient you. This is a view through the abdomen. Imagine that the subject's body is going right through this page, with his head and chest toward you and his feet poking out the other side. If we cut him in half, this CAT scan view is what we would see. (Think of the kind of slice we make in a tree when we count the age rings).

The light grey material in this scan is fat. As you can see, a considerable layer of fat sits outside the body wall and goes around the entire body circumference. This is the fat you can grab with your hands; better known as

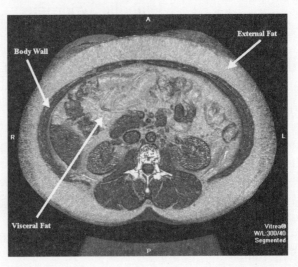

the "pot belly" or "love handles." As I said earlier, this outer fat, while unsightly, is relatively harmless. But now, look inside the body. The dark spots are internal organs. The mass of grey gunk, deposited everywhere around them, is visceral fat. That's dangerous stuff.

Large amounts of fatty tissue have no business being inside the belly. Internal fat smothers important body organs like the liver, pancreas, and intestines and can even invade the organs themselves.

This unwanted fatty mess causes real problems. The core of the body is an important business center where vital jobs are performed. It should be clean and free-flowing, not packed with blubber.

Internal belly fat gives off dangerous inflammatory chemicals with names like tumor necrosis factor and interleukin-6. Secreted right at a major interchange on the vascular highway, these bad actors can get directly into the blood stream. The result is inflammation throughout the body. Inflammatory changes damage the arteries, making them prone to blockage. When vessels block off, a heart attack, stroke or other vascular event follows.

Inflammation also appears to provoke cancers. The inflammatory chemicals made by visceral fat may explain why obese people are at risk for so many malignancies, including cancers of the kidney, uterus, breast, colon, gall bladder, and thyroid. In 2002, cancers linked to obesity represented 14 percent of all new cancers diagnosed in men, and a whopping 51 percent of all new cancers diagnosed in women..

Metabolic Syndrome:
A Confusing Name for the Newest American Epidemic

Sadly, a marked increase in inflammation is only the beginning of the problem with visceral fat. Far greater numbers of overweight people are affected by an even more destructive consequence of the large belly, a condition called Metabolic Syndrome.

This syndrome is a group of linked medical problems. It occurs when visceral fat creates problems with insulin, one of the body's most vital hormones.

Because an insulin problem is at the heart of metabolic syndrome, I think a more accurate name is "Struggling Insulin Syndrome." As you read on, you may notice that I use both names.

The Components of Struggling Insulin Syndrome (Metabolic Syndrome):

1. Waist size greater than 35" in a woman and 40" in a man.
2. Triglyceride levels of over 150.
3. Good cholesterol (HDL) levels of less than 50 in a woman, less than 40 in a man.
4. Blood pressure of greater than 130/85.
5. Fasting blood sugar of greater than 100.

Three of these components must be present to make the diagnosis.

Understanding the nature of Struggling Insulin Syndrome requires a bit of mini-medical school, but I hope you'll indulge me. Since insulin is what is affected, let's begin with reviewing what insulin does in the first place.

Insulin is a hormone produced by a small organ called the pancreas. Most people know it as the hormone that controls blood sugar, and that is indeed one of its major jobs.

Every element that travels in the blood is controlled within a tight range by the body. Sugar traveling in the blood is no different. Insulin is in charge of keeping those sugar levels within a certain range.

High levels of blood sugar are damaging to your blood vessels. Once sugar starts rising in the bloodstream, the body calls on insulin immediately. Insulin's job is to find somewhere else to put the sugar. That will lower blood levels to an acceptable range.

To give you an idea of how little sugar normally travels in the blood, you may be surprised to learn that the amount of sugar in your entire bloodstream right now (assuming you're not diabetic) is equal to the contents of one of those small sugar packets you put in your coffee (one teaspoon or four grams).

Sugar levels in the blood go up after you eat sugary foods. Importantly, they also rise when you eat starches, because starches turn into sugar during digestion. It doesn't take much to imagine how frequently our blood sugar rises. Starches and sugars dominate the American diet.

Separated at Birth? The "S" Foods

Most people have observed that starchy foods and sugars make them fat. This is no coincidence. Starch and sugar are twins; just two different forms of the same thing. Let's call them the "S Foods." Starchy foods like bread, pasta, rice, cereal, grains and potatoes are made up of basic sugar molecules that are strung together to form bigger chains. Sugars, on the other hand, are made up of one or two basic molecules alone.

To imagine this, think of plain sugar as simple wooden blocks. Bread, pasta, potatoes, rice, flour, cereals, whole grains and other starches are just large, varied shapes built from these blocks. You may build a skyscraper, a train or a circus wagon, but when you break each creation down, you will still be left with the same pile of blocks on the table.

Sugar is one of a number of fuels your body can use (proteins and fats are others). In order to get sugar to each cell, the body uses the bloodstream as a transport system. In the blood, S Foods are carried in their simplest form—the basic block. Your digestive system is given the job of breaking down those large starch molecules. Since sugars and starches are made up of the same basic blocks, the two are identical once digestion gets through with them. Shortly after you eat S Foods, both enter the blood as exactly the same thing: blood sugar. (Figure 1)

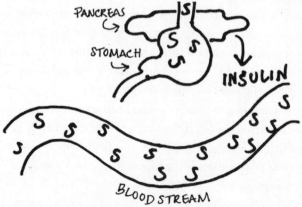

Figure 1

Pretty much everyone knows that eating a lot of sugar isn't a good idea. I have never met anyone who would consider pouring cups of sugar into their coffee, yet the same folks have no problem eating pounds of starch. People make this error only because they don't realize that the two are the same. Now, you are armed with important information: when you eat starch, you eat sugar. For a lot more information about S Foods and how they gained such a foothold in our diet, be sure to read Chapter Seven, which is devoted solely to them.

Insulin Gets a Call

The body is made up of billions of cells, each working diligently. A particularly busy group of cells, though, are those found in your muscles. These cells are like little factories, working actively and frequently calling for fuel. A new supply is constantly delivered by the bloodstream to keep the machinery going.

After you eat an S Food and it is torn apart, the resulting sugar passes into the blood and sugar levels rise. As you'll remember, insulin controls these levels, so a call for insulin is soon issued.

Insulin functions as a kind of foreman. In order to get sugar out of the bloodstream, it diverts it toward muscular factories. Once there, insulin opens closed cell doors with a special key. The sugar then passes inside where it is burned as fuel (Figure 2).

Insulin's Second Job

Things are never simple in the body. Insulin turns out to have a second job that most people don't know about. In addition to controlling blood sugar levels, insulin is also responsible for storing fat.

In order to perform this second job, insulin accesses a second key, opens up the body's fat cells and sends part of the excess sugar their way.

Once inside fat cells, the sugar is converted to fat and tucked away for a rainy day (Figure 2).

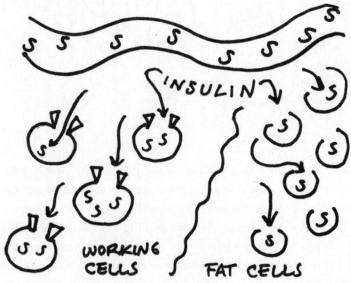

Figure 2

Key Failure!

(Everything I've described so far is part of our normal design. Something goes very wrong, though, when our bellies get clogged with fat. These oily, yellow deposits throw a monkey wrench into our precisely calibrated machinery.)

For reasons that are still unclear, internal belly fat causes muscle key failure. When insulin attempts to clear sugar from the blood by putting it into muscle cells, the cell doors refuse to open. Insulin's muscle key seems to be out of order. The great irony, though, is that insulin's fat cell key still works just fine!

The insulin foreman still has a job to do and that is to lower blood sugar. With muscle cells stuck tight, the only way to get rid of the sugar is to send a flood of it into fat storage (Figure 3).

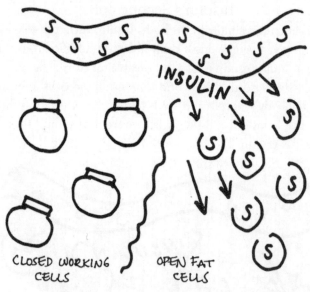

CLOSED WORKING CELLS   OPEN FAT CELLS

Figure 3

Doctors call this state of affairs "insulin resistance," but it is more accurate to call it "partial insulin resistance" because only the muscle cells resist insulin's key. Fat cells remain quite able to take up sugar.

In insulin resistant people, fat cells get fatter and fatter while muscle cells remain locked and underfed. The two simply can't help each other out. Some have speculated that the extreme hunger described by overweight people may come from the fact that their working cells are "starving" and sending anxious messages to the brain. In the meantime, the rest of their body looks anything but starved.

In order to satisfy this persistent hunger, most people choose S Foods. You can see where this is going. S Foods break down into sugar. The muscle cells are closed, so the sugar is diverted to fat. The expanding fat makes the muscle problem worse. It's a vicious cycle, something that your body desperately wants to overcome. But how?

The Less than Perfect Solution

The body comes up with a single solution. It asks the pancreas to churn out lots of insulin (what I call "Big Insulin"), hoping that massive amounts of the stuff will overwhelm those stubbornly closed cell doors. Perhaps if insulin carries a billy club it can pummel those muscle cells into opening. (Figure 4)

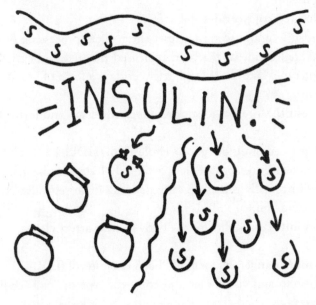

Figure 4

This solution works for a time. Big Insulin is a bully that intimidates the cell doors into cracking open and the situation may stabilize for a few months or a few years. But at a cost to you. The insulin foreman was once a nice quiet guy, going about his rounds. Now he is a huge, overwhelming presence. Your perfectly balanced system was not built to deal with these hulking amounts of insulin. Like bullies everywhere, Big Insulin is toxic.

How Big Insulin Makes You Pay

Once Big Insulin and visceral fat get together, you are well on your way to the complete Struggling Insulin Syndrome. Together, these two bad guys cooperate to severely injury your cardiovascular system. They do this by partnering to create a number of harmful outcomes:

1. Inflammatory chemicals in the blood

As you learned earlier, visceral fat manufactures these.

The result? Inflammatory damage to vessel walls.

2. High blood pressure

Big Insulin is a constricting agent and it tightens blood vessels. As vessels clamp down, blood pressure goes up.

The result? Vessel walls that are further damaged by being battered at high pressure.

3. Elevated triglycerides

Big Insulin and visceral fat reset the normal processing of cholesterol and triglyceride in the liver. Increased production of triglyceride is one outcome. Like cholesterol, triglyceride is a form of blood fat that can clog arteries.

The result? More fats to stick to damaged vessels and form clogs.

4. Depressed levels of "good" cholesterol (HDL)

The same liver reset causes less "good" cholesterol to be made. HDL cholesterol normally cleans up fatty deposits in vessel walls. Now you don't have enough.

The result? Less ability for the body to clear artery clogs.

5. A more dangerous form of "bad" cholesterol (LDL)

Big Insulin and visceral fat also affect the type of "bad" cholesterol (LDL) your body makes. Bad cholesterol can be packaged into large, fluffy particles that are relatively harmless to vessel walls. Now, however, production is now shifted toward smaller, more irritating particles. This small, dense form of LDL can insinuate itself into cracks and other damaged areas in vessel walls starting off the process that leads to blockage.

The result? Small LDL particles can lodge in walls damaged by inflammation and high blood pressure. This is a set up for heart attack, stroke, and other vascular disease.

6. Elevated blood sugar

As Struggling Insulin Syndrome is developing, blood sugar may stay normal for a time. This is because Big Insulin is straining to get sugar into the cells and keep blood sugar from rising. This tenuous situation is known as "pre-diabetes." Those with pre-diabetes may be completely unaware of it. Only their pancreas~ churning out Big Insulin day after day ~is aware of how hard it is working. Eventually, the pancreas starts to lose the battle and sugar backs up into the blood.

The result? Elevated sugar levels or actual diabetes.

Back to the Source

Time to go all the way back to our CAT scan. It was visceral fat that started this whole process rolling. Visceral fat, then, is what we must seek to treat. Significant weight loss can eliminate this fat which, in turn, reverses insulin resistance. Insulin's key starts to open cellular doors again and the need for bullying levels of insulin disappears. The pancreas can finally rest.

But let's say the problem is ignored. Insulin continues to be made at high levels and the struggling pancreas becomes severely overworked. Eventually its insulin producing cells burn out like a smoking piece of machinery. The pancreas fails.

When insulin production drops off, or fails completely, there is no way for sugar to get out of the blood. Swarms of glucose molecules soon overwhelm the blood stream and spill out in the urine. Take a blood test, and it reads 150, 300, even 500...this is called adult onset diabetes.

Some diabetics continue to make small amounts of insulin and can get by with pills that help boost production and sensitivity. Others have complete burnout. Since no one can live entirely without insulin, final burn-out means that permanent treatment with injected insulin is inevitable.

A Little Sugar in the Blood

Diabetes has become so common in our world that many of us see it as a trivial annoyance, easily treated with medication. Many of my patients tell me in an offhand way that they have "a little sugar in the blood." But here's the problem, by the time doctors note sugar going up, your body has likely been silently struggling for years with staggering loads of pancreatic work. "I have a little sugar" actually might better translate to "I smell a little smoke" —the burning smell of your pancreas beginning its meltdown.

When you detect fire, it only makes sense to run for the first exit. In this case, that's an immediate exit from current dietary habits and a brisk loss of weight. If you make those changes stick, chances are good that you can salvage your health.

No one should underestimate diabetes, which is a debilitating and destructive disease. Normally, the body works hard to keep sugar levels controlled in the blood for a very good reason. When unchecked, that syrupy sugar destroys blood vessels. As you have already learned, these vessels are the vital transportation corridors of your body. It's terribly important that you keep them smooth, open and flowing. More than that, blood vessels exist in every part of you, so diabetes has the potential to destroy everything, most notably your eyes, your kidneys, and your heart.

Most people have observed that starchy foods and sugars make them fat. This is no coincidence. Starch and sugar are twins; just two different forms of the same thing.

If we add diabetes to the burden of inflamed vessels, high cholesterol, and triglycerides and the daily pounding of high blood pressure that make up Struggling Insulin Syndrome, we can see that allowing this multiple threat is like taking a large mallet to your perfectly designed physiology.

Having Struggling Insulin Syndrome triples your risk of coronary artery disease, heart attack, and stroke. It quadruples your risk of dying from any cause and gives you six times the risk of dying from a cardiac incident.

The majority of patients I take care of have Struggling Insulin Syndrome, yet few have been made aware of their diagnosis. Worse, they have no idea that their visceral fat is directly causing most of their medical problems. This is information that is vitally important for POWs. Weight regain will restart this cycle.

Metabolic Syndrome (Struggling Insulin Syndrome) is shockingly common. The current prevalence in American adults is believed to be around 27 percent—greater than one out of four of us! Some groups, like Hispanic women, have rates as high as 37 percent. Older people have higher rates, too. By age sixty to sixty-nine, the syndrome is found in nearly 45 percent of us.

As Baby Boomers get older, we are facing an epidemic of Struggling Insulin Syndrome related disease. Can you imagine the outcry if we were to learn that one in four American adults had cancer?

The number of Americans with cancers as of 2003 was 3.6 percent. That's four out of 100. Yet twenty-seven out of 100 have Metabolic Syndrome, a highly dangerous condition that is costing our society billions of health care dollars.

Break the String

I ask my patients to visualize Metabolic or Struggling Insulin Syndrome as an unattractive necklace made up of a series of heavy beads. To make this necklace, circle your waist with a string. This string represents the fat around your middle. Onto this string you can thread a bead for high blood pressure, one for high triglycerides, one for low good cholesterol, one for elevated inflammation, one for high total cholesterol, and a big heavy one for elevated blood sugar. Your necklace may have more beads than one person's and fewer than another's. Either way, it is heavy, ugly, and unwanted. So take off the weight and break the string! Getting rid of the visceral fat makes all the beads fall away.

Having broken the string, you must prevent your body from ever re-entering the jewelry business. You will have to work diligently to avoid rebuilding your visceral fat. This is the job you are learning to do by reading this book. Your new, lower weight is more of a gift than you ever imagined. Now that you have been warned about the dangers of regaining that weight, let's turn our attention to what we can do to keep you right where you are today.

Chapter Wrap

- Excess fat, particularly around the middle of your body is *not* harmless.
- Even if you have never had an abnormal blood test, you are better off maintaining your new low weight than gaining any of it back.
- If you previously suffered from elevated blood sugar, high blood pressure, cholesterol or triglyceride problems and these have improved with weight loss, you have made huge inroads into creating a new, healthy body.
- Don't be fooled into underestimating the dangers of fat simply because so many around you are overweight.
- Consider your future and do things today that will insure health tomorrow.

Chapter Four

A Body Built for Lean Times

Eat food, not too much, mostly plants. That, more or less, is the short answer to the supposedly incredibly complicated and confusing question of what we humans should eat...
                    —Michael Pollan, *In Defense of Food*

The very nature of our bodies suggests that humans were designed for lean times. Until very recently, our ancestors were unsure of a steady food supply and the search for sustenance was man's primary occupation. Ancient peoples faced frequent periods of deprivation—even starvation. Since this state of affairs persisted for millions of years, a body design slowly developed which perfectly matched the challenges of this environment.

This is not surprising. Observation tells us that living creatures develop in response to the conditions in which they live. Frogs live both in water and on land and can breathe in either environment at different times in their life cycle. Humans, on the other hand, have lungs solely for breathing air. For millions of years we have lived on land and our bodies have tailored themselves to this life. Unlike the frog, we are helpless if we fall in the drink.

Our body design reflects a greater than two-million-year experience with scarce (and particular) food supplies. As a result, we have abundant mechanisms for supporting us through starvation, but lack good equipment for submersion in an ocean of food.

Our long experience with eating in a scarce environment has encouraged our bodies to create any number of fat-enabling hormones. In an uncertain food world it is good to store fat whenever possible. We humans appear to have learned this lesson well. This ancient mechanism remains a part of our body blueprint, a trait which geneticist James Neel called the "thrifty gene." While there is still debate about the existence of such a gene, there is no debating the fact that the majority of us store fat avidly when modern food is plentiful.

When you overeat—especially the S Foods (grains, starches, sugars)—your body is unprepared. As you just learned, the insulin system is poorly suited for constant demands. In time, an over-reliance on this fragile hormone leads to the Struggling Insulin Syndrome and, often, type 2 diabetes.

If you doubt how easily insulin can get us into trouble in our modern world, you need only look at recent diabetes statistics. The number of new cases of adult onset diabetes has risen 100 percent since the 1970s. One out of every ten people in their forties and fifties is currently diabetic; in those sixty and older, the figure is a startling one in five. By 2050, the number of diabetic Americans is expected to rise from 11 million to 29 million. Most startling of all is the prediction by some researchers that one out of three Americans born in the year 2000 will develop diabetes in their lifetime.

We must ask ourselves why this dangerous epidemic is occurring with such rapidity. Our genes and bodies remain the same as they always were. If nothing has changed in our biology, the cause must be a rapidly changing environment. The fact that the diabetes epidemic results from lifestyle issues makes it a double tragedy. Not only are millions losing their limbs, kidneys, eyesight, and lives, but their suffering could have been avoided. We won't be able to move a step closer to prevention, though, until we take an honest look at the increasingly destructive food environment that surrounds us.

Our bodies do better with fewer S Foods. But it may also turn out that our bodies are better adapted to eating less food of any type.

Numerous studies of many species (including worms, fish, flies, and rats) confirm that insect and animal life can actually be extended if calories are reduced over the lifespan. Calorically restricted animals not only live longer, but also maintain a more youthful appearance and vigor. In addition, scientists at the National Institute on Aging contend that excess calories are a major risk factor for a number of age-related diseases, including cardiovascular disease, type 2 diabetes, Alzheimer's disease, and Parkinson's disease.

When you choose not to eat for several hours, think of yourself as a one-way street with the arrow flipped in the "Release Fat" direction.

How much calorie restriction is enough? And does it work in humans? We are unlikely to know the answer in the near future. To find out whether caloric restriction works to extend life, we will need to bide our time until current human subjects become old. This is a long time to wait, particularly for those of us already in our fifties and more.

Who are the human subjects we will look to? Many are part of a group called the CRON movement, an acronym which stands for "Caloric Restriction with Optimal Nutrition." CRON practitioners follow very restricted diets and are often extremely lean. It is important to note that because they consume so little, they choose only foods with the highest nutritional value—the "optimal nutrition" part.

While we can't yet comment on their longevity, results from some shorter-term studies of CRON practitioners show benefits. Lean subjects who eat approximately 1800 calories a day for about six years have many markers of excellent health. Heart function, for example, is reported to be equivalent to that of people sixteen years younger. While these studies are not perfect, they do suggest that people who eat less seem to be healthier than their free-eating counterparts. When looking at this data it is important to remember that CRON practitioners, while eating small amounts of food, eat a highly nutritious selection. It is always possible that it is the content of the calories rather than the amount that makes the difference in their health.

While initial studies look promising, the long-term safety of caloric restriction remains unknown. Dr. Roy Walford was one of CRON's earliest and most devoted practitioners. Dr. Walford researched and wrote a number of books on human caloric restriction and practiced a CRON lifestyle for many years. He was also a part of the Biosphere team, a 1990s experiment in which eight scientists lived in a completely closed environment for two years.

Unfortunately, Dr. Walford did not reach the extreme longevity he hoped for but died of Lou Gehrig's disease (amyotrophic lateral sclerosis) at age seventy-nine. Might the onset of this neurodegenerative disease have been related to his CRON lifestyle? Dr. Walford felt that his disease came from environmental problems that occurred within the Biosphere, but no one can be sure. While an active CRON community, including Dr. Walford's daughter, continue to swear by the CRON approach, the jury remains out on extreme caloric restriction.

Whether or not you believe in the promise of CRON, you can adapt some of its principles to your life as a weight maintainer. It seems reasonable to conclude that the body is taxed by various byproducts of overeating and that we are likely designed to do best when we eat less. Rather than starve ourselves, though, we can eat judiciously and scarcely.

If we accept that we must create our own version of food scarcity to stay healthy, we need a plan for making it all work. I have found that for most maintainers, the best way to eat scarcely is to follow three principles:

1. Eat one major meal per day.
2. Spend some portions of the day in the non-eating state.
3. Make all food choices highly nutritious.

Explaining the Three Principles

Principle One: Eat one major meal per day

Eating one complete meal daily is one of the 12 Tough Rules; you can read more about it in Section Two. In recent years, many have questioned our American practice of eating three square meals a day. Some have suggested that we "graze" continually, others that we eat a certain number of small meals per day. The confusion is understandable. In the past, when we worked physically and vigorously it made sense to eat solid meals at particular intervals. For farmers who rose with the sun, a large breakfast came after several hours of early work. Midday meals also reflected the need to refuel tired muscles. But as you well know, our environment has changed. Do we still need large meals eaten at 7, 12, and 6? Our steadily increasing size tells us that we need to find more creative ways of eating for health in the modern era.

I have found that maintainers do very nicely when they program themselves for one meal. This does not mean that they only eat once a day, but that they allow themselves only one complete meal. It remains important to eat smaller amounts at other times—what I call "Mini-Meals" and "Fast Grabs." On the other hand, expecting only one major meal in their day gets them in the habit of food scheduling.

To do this, look ahead at the beginning of each day. If you will be going out to dinner, lunch is liable to be some fruit and nuts, or a low fat yogurt and a salad. Some people do better having their larger meal at lunchtime and eating sparingly at dinner. You may choose to alternate the placement of your one major meal depending on the day—lunch one day, dinner the next. This is perfectly fine. What should that major meal look like? You will find a detailed description in Rule 6, Section Two.

Principle Two: Flip the arrow: spend parts of the day in the non-eating state

The hormones that work to break down fat and glycogen (stored sugar), need to be left alone to do their work. I believe that the American habit of continual grazing leads to a greater tendency to store fat.

Think of the body's fat processing mechanism as a one-way street. As you learned in Chapter Three, when insulin is turned on, fat cells are open, storage is occurring, and what is put into the fat cells is trapped inside. When eating stops and insulin declines, the opposing hormones take over, fat is free to move out of the cells and breakdown can occur.

Give your body a chance to regroup. Eat and then stop eating. When you choose not to eat for several hours, think of yourself as a one-way street with the arrow flipped in the "Release Fat" direction. Each of us can do perfectly well with a couple of hours each day that don't involve eating something. Think about it. In today's world, how often do such food-free periods occur?

To flip your arrow, physically remove yourself from the eating environment, whether that is your kitchen or the place in your office where food is kept. Try to spend an hour or two after eating without eating again. This is not a hard and fast rule, but a good habit. Learn to enjoy the subtle pleasure of feeling light, not full. Most of my patients describe enjoying this feeling during dieting and maintenance. Being pleasantly empty is not an intense rush, but neither does it have to be something to be avoided.

Principle Three: Make all food choices highly nutritious

Just as those who follow the CRON diet make the most out of every morsel, so should you. The worst thing you can do for your body is to eat scarcely and poorly. So make it a habit to evaluate whatever goes into your mouth. Honor the miracle that is your body by feeding it only what it needs and that which is high quality.

The temptation to eat scarcely and poorly is a particular concern for patients who have had bariatric surgery. Without proper dietary counseling, it is easy for someone who must eat small amounts to consume nothing but tiny bites of candy, ice cream, and French fries. Remember that starvation does not only refer to calories. It is perfectly possible to starve your body of vital nutrients while eating large amounts of food, a situation that has become only too common in today's world.

To make nutritious food choices, simply follow the ancient diet guidelines that are discussed in the next two chapters. If you eat the foods your genes are programmed to recognize, you will automatically get the proper balance of fiber, micronutrients, vitamins, minerals, and good and bad fats. All this without counting, calculation, or concern.

Chapter Wrap

- Remove your body from modern eating by creating your own version of a scarce food environment.
- Do this by relying on one major meal per day, supplemented by two smaller Mini-Meals and some Fast Grabs. (See the 12 Tough Rules to learn more.)
- Follow Primarian eating guidelines (Chapters Five and Six) when choosing your foods.
- Spend at least several hours of each day in a non-eating state, letting your body use up some of its stores.

Chapter Five

Eating With Your Genes:
Becoming a Primarian

Living organisms thrive best in the milieu and on the diet to which they were evolutionarily adapted; this is a fundamental axiom of biology.
  —James O'Keefe, M.D. and Loren Cordain, Ph.D.

In the last chapter we discussed that humans are best adapted to a particular eating style—one that our bodies have come to know over endless time. In this chapter, we'll discuss that diet more specifically and learn how its consumption can bring our lives back in line with our genetic expectations. Doing this is critical, both for health and for maintaining lost weight.

Some years ago, a lightbulb went off in my head regarding ancient eating. At the time, I foolishly supposed that I was alone in figuring out what seemed to be the simplest and most elegant solution for health: a return to some version of the ancient diet. I was completely wrong. As I started to read and research, I discovered that many experts in paleonutrition had been championing such a diet for years. Two scientists in particular, Dr. S. Boyd Eaton and Dr. Loren Cordain, have done exhaustive research into the disharmony between our bodies and the diets we currently eat. They have written elegantly on the subject as well. Much of what you will read in this chapter and the next is based on their work and that of others who support "paleolithic" eating. Should you want a more extensive treatment of the rationale and research behind their thinking, I refer you to their excellent works, listed in the resource section at the back of this book.

> *As our world becomes more complex, our eating style needs to return to its origins, bringing us back into harmony with our ancient design.*

Refuse to Regain!

We live in a wonderful era in which eradication of infections, improvements in sanitation, and the marvels of modern medicine have created longer lives than ever before. While our recent longevity is undeniably positive, our modern way of life has allowed new problems to emerge. As we live longer, we find ourselves plagued by chronic diseases—conditions which occur mostly as the consequence of years of inactivity and poor eating. Imagine the power over health we might have if we could combine a perfect eating plan with all of the advances of modern medical technology.

In fact, this is precisely the unprecedented opportunity available to us in the 21st century. We can live long lives through optimal nutrition and exercise, and then have our older years enhanced by technologies such as joint replacement, cataract surgery, and cochlear implants. While modern food supplies give us access to broad affordable nutrition, science adds the ability to shore up body parts that weaken with age. Marrying these two technologies can allow us to live long—yet remain vital. While there will always be a limit to the length of our years, we can hope to be well throughout most of them.

My own father is a prime example. After suffering a heart attack at age fifty, he completely revamped his diet and began a daily exercise regimen. This kept him in good shape for over forty years. At age ninety-four, he was able to have an aortic aneurysm repaired with a modern, non-invasive technique. He has also benefited from a pacemaker and modern treatments for macular degeneration. But he has only been able to enjoy the results of these technologies because of the underlying health he began to create years ago through diet and activity. He continues to live actively, travels with my mother (who as of this writing is eighty-nine), and reads *The New York Times* front to back.

While scientists can be relied upon to create new bionic parts and hi-tech supports, it remains up to us to figure out the optimal diet. Luckily, the solution is simplicity itself. As our world becomes more complex, our eating style needs to return to its origins, bringing us back into harmony with our ancient design.

The strategy that I advocate derives from a most basic principle: eat what nature intended you to eat and nothing else. I call this diet a "Primarian" eating plan, meaning a diet consisting mostly of the primary or original foods our ancient ancestors consumed. I will describe this concept in greater detail in this chapter and the next. As you will soon see, our bodies are machines that know how to run on very particular fuels, fuels we have largely abandoned. Once you understand why we function as we do, the rules of eating will fall easily into place.

Why an Ancient Diet?

Ask any five-year-old the following question: "If someone gave you a lion to take care of, what would you feed it?" Even a kindergartener can tell you that the answer is raw meat. Each one of us respects the ancient lineage of lions. We also understand intuitively that, over millennia, nature has designed a certain diet for wild creatures. A lion will die if he gives up meat for bagels. Despite this basic understanding, we don't connect with the fact that we humans are just like lions—ancient beings with a noble heritage and diet needs dictated by the natural world.

The importance of eating what nature designed seems obvious to those who take care of animals. Zoo nutrition is based on finding diets that closely match the needs of animals who normally live in the wild. Sometimes, even the most carefully crafted approximations won't do. Koala populations, for example, need to eat a special diet of eucalyptus leaves. They can only be kept in habitats that can provide regular access to this food.

The benefits of ancient diet have also not been lost on small animal owners who are facing a growing problem with obesity in pets. Dog owners may be aware of the Bones and Raw Food (BARF) movement, which advocates feeding pets foods that look a lot more like what their wild ancestors ate. According to Ian Billinghurst, the Australian veterinarian who is a voice of this movement:

> Artificial grain based dog foods cause innumerable health problems. They are not what your dog was programmed to eat during its long process of evolution. A biologically appropriate diet for a dog is one that consists of raw whole foods similar to those eaten by the dogs' wild ancestors.

The eating of original diets, then, seems to make sense for animals. But does the ancient, or Primarian concept translate to humans? I believe it does. Our ancestors, the Hominid species, emerged 2.6 million years ago and spent hundreds of thousands of years eating particular food types. Like the lion, your genes know this diet and expect it. They developed programs in response to this diet which are still a part of your hard-wiring.

Genes are the master managers of body operations. Therefore, each of us carries a management manual written hundreds of thousands of years ago. It's still a good manual. The problem is that the directions within expect the world to look pretty much the way it did when the manual was written. Unfortunately, things have changed a good deal. Enormous alterations in our diet have left our genes baffled. We are like the bagel-eating lion, suffering the dire consequences of eating outside of our genetic comfort zone.

But Food Is Food, Isn't It?

We human beings tend to forget that we are part of the natural world. Because we are omnivores—both plant and meat eaters—we have grown accustomed to think of ourselves as being able to eat just about anything. We also believe that most foods are equivalent—all simply different forms of fuel. Given what we know of the dietary needs of other living things, that belief doesn't make sense.

Here's a simple example from the inanimate world: imagine that your house is heated by natural gas. The price climbs, so you decide to pour heating oil into the gas furnace. Ridiculous, right? Whether it's kerosene, wood, or lumps of coal, the wrong fuel will turn your furnace into a worthless piece of scrap metal. The fact that these substances are all fuels is immaterial. The question is: does the fuel match the machine?

Your house runs on a particular kind of fuel. So does the lion. Is it so hard to believe that human beings were designed to run on certain kinds of fuel, too? A poor fuel choice can cause your own machinery to become mightily gummed up. In the body, these messy conditions turn out to be clogged arteries, pounds of unhealthy belly fat, and unwanted sugar polluting the blood stream.

OK, so our fuels have changed; haven't our genes kept up?

Most of us know enough about science to know that our genes can mutate or mold themselves to new conditions. Unfortunately for our modern eating habits, these changes can take tens of thousands, even millions of years. In fact, your entire library of genes—inherited from your ancient forebears—has barely changed over the past 40,000 years. We now know that except for about .02 percent of their function, your genes look exactly the same as did those of your Stone Age ancestors.

Adaptation to new foods can occur, but it's an incredibly slow process. Let's look at one example—the ability to digest cow's milk. As you will soon learn, animal milk is rather new on the human menu, first appearing a mere 10,000 years ago. Prior to this time, milk was a food for infants and came solely in the human version—from Mom. To break down the milk, our genetic script called for us to make an enzyme called lactase in infancy. The script then shut down production of this enzyme in early childhood, around the time of weaning. This tiny program, designed millions of years ago, is the reason that as many as 70 percent of today's world population are lactose intolerant. Simply put, lactose intolerant adults lack the enzyme to digest milk because it was "appropriately" shut off when they were toddlers. Their operating manual is blissfully unaware of the invention of whipped cream, gelato, and mozzarella.

In those who can digest milk, the trait has taken somewhere in the neighborhood of 250 generations (5000 years) to become established. This is a very long time. Furthermore, lactose tolerance isn't a true mutation. It is actually an example of neoteny, the persistence into adulthood of a gene trait we already possessed as children.

Human genes can change, but only over millennia. Mutation or not, given the time span required for the body to change its food programming, it is undoubtedly vain to hope that we can adapt to unending loads of potatoes, pasta, cake, and bread in the very near future.

What Is the Ancient Diet? A Brief History of Eating

I said earlier that eating Primarian meant eating what nature intended and nothing else. But what did nature intend? That is not always easy to sort out. Let's take a stab at figuring this out by looking at the history of human eating. Our food consumption has gone through three distinct stages.

Stage One, primary foods:
What you can hunt, pick, fish, or gather

For almost all of human history, our ancestors were hunter-gatherers, tribal people who roamed the earth eating what they could hunt, fish, pick, and gather. Our hunter-gatherer years began long before civilization and agriculture came into being. They covered a vast time span that started in the Paleolithic period 2.5 million years ago and persisted until just 10,000 years ago. This was the period of ancient eating; the foods we became accustomed to during these years make up the bulk of the

Primarian diet. The relationship between 2.5 million years and 10,000 years is not easy to conceptualize but one thing is certain—10,000 years is a microflash in our developmental timeframe.

Here is an easy reference. If man's entire existence is imagined as one day (and each hour of that day equals 100,000 years of actual time), humans were hunter-gatherers for every moment except the final six minutes. This enormous time disparity means that our genes have had endless time to accommodate to hunter-gatherer, or Primarian foods, and no time at all to adapt to recent additions. Which foods are specifically Primarian? They are the original products of the earth and its animals.

An easy way to figure out which foods are primary is to imagine yourself forced to survive in a nearby national park. What could you eat if you absolutely could not leave its boundaries? First, you could find a variety of lean animals meats such as deer, rabbit, possum, and squirrel (don't panic, there's no squirrel or possum on this diet, but lean meats of any type are fine). There would also be poultry, perhaps even wild turkeys, duck, and quail. The eggs of these birds could be found in their nests. Fish may be caught. If your park system borders an ocean, a variety of shellfish and seafood would be available to you. Although today's park-goer might be unfamiliar with which plants are edible, there would certainly be a wide array of vegetable matter and an assortment of fruits. Nuts and berries, the seeds of a few wild grasses, and some roots would round out the picture.

These primary foods make up the diet that is most familiar to your ancient core. The rationale is simple: since we can't change the way our genes see food, why not change our diet to match our genes?

Fortunately, the Primarian diet is easily replicated in any supermarket or restaurant. Lean meats, poultry, fish and other seafood, eggs, vegetables, fruits, nuts, and berries form the menu.

Of course, there are some differences between modern versions of primary foods and their ancient cousins (that squirrel, for example). The grain-fed meats we eat today are a lot less lean than the meat of animals which grazed and ran wild, so we need to be careful to limit fatty cuts of meat and to minimize the fatty skin of poultry. Ancient vegetables and fruits would have been smaller and more fibrous than our modern varieties, meaning that today's sugary cultivated fruits like pineapples and bananas should be eaten sparingly. Nevertheless, a good rule of thumb is to eat the types of foods that you could eat if stranded in the woods.

The simple components of our original human diet stand in stark contrast to those elements that are missing: particularly the ubiquitous and fattening S Foods. You already know the S Foods as the sugars and starches that dominate our modern diet, but these starches and sugars, even in their most basic form, were not part of our original menu.

The first missing element is sugar. With the exception of the modest sugar in fruits, simple sugar was found only in honey. Honey gathering was unlikely to be a daily occurrence and was only successful when hunter-gatherers managed to outwit the bees.

While sugary foods were rare, their occasional appearance provided a valuable source of bankable calories for ancients living from meal to meal. To make sure we'd eat sugar calories when they were available, it appears we have been designed to like sweet things very much. The desire for sugar, most likely important for survival in the ancient world, seems to be the origin of our modern sweet tooth.

The second missing element in the Primarian diet is starch. As you already know, starch is simply a bigger molecular form of sugar. It is found in tubers (potatoes), in grains (wheat, rye, oats, corn, rice, etc.) and in the products of these foods—especially the flours, breads, cereals, and pastas created from them. Starches are the king of the modern diet, yet when we look at the Diet-in-the-Park, we are hard pressed to find them.

Isn't bread the "staff of life?" Although we tend to think of grain and the bread made from it as very ancient, a brief look around our park shows us that fields of large edible grains don't grow wild and were therefore unavailable to your ancient forebears. The absence of grain means that flour, breads and cereals were not a part of the original diet.

Grains that do grow wild are found in the form of wild grasses. The small seeds of these plants were difficult for ancient people to harvest and even harder to eat. Paleonutritionists have observed that ancient people ate these seeds mainly under starvation conditions. In fact, no other primate eats grain in the wild.

Large baking potatoes don't grow wild, nor do most beans, soy and other legumes. And what about a third missing element—dairy? During our hunter-gatherer days, humans did not keep domesticated animals and did not milk. Mother's milk was our only milk exposure.

Despite all these missing pieces, research indicates that ancients ate well. Diet composition changed seasonally depending on the plant and animal material available; fossil evidence suggests that many different types of foods were generally consumed. Some cultures ate only animal foods, others were vegetarian—but all ate directly from the earth.

Stage Two, newcomer foods:
Grains, legumes, and dairy

Then, about 10,000 years ago, a massive shift in the human diet occurred. Humans learned how to farm. Farming meant that our ancestors discovered how to grow larger and more usable grains from seeds and how to keep animals in flocks. The growing of grain appears to have begun in the Middle East with the cultivation of weeds and wild grasses. About 1,000 years later, rice was cultivated in China and corn in Central America. Cultivation of potatoes and beans also appeared during this period. Domestication of animals brought milk into the diet. Since these foods were very new to human history, we'll refer to them as "Newcomer Foods:"

Grains:	Wheat, rye, corn, oats, barley, etc.
Legumes:	Beans, soy, peanuts, peas, lentils
Tubers:	Potatoes, yams, starchy root plants
Animal milk:	Cow, goat, and others

The advent of farming was a crucial step in human history. Once our ancestors learned how to produce grain, a ready source of calories became available right outside the front door. The addition of flocks of animals and the milk and meat they produced allowed man to stop chasing his prey, settle down, and turn his attention to building communities and ultimately civilization.

While no one can deny the vital role agriculture played in human development, the resulting dietary change had consequences. As our ancestors stopped hunting and gathering, they became shorter. Osteoporosis and other bone problems developed, as well as dental cavities and vitamin deficiencies. This may have reflected decreased nutrition in the grain-based diet or the fact that wide-ranging foods were no longer consumed. Whatever the case, our diet shifted greatly to a dependence on grains and legumes—foods which provide fiber and a number of nutrients, but combine them with a large dose of starchy carbohydrate.

Stage Three, altered foods:
The foods made by machines

Altered Foods are those food products we have created since machines came to the fore in the late 1800s. In 1937, the great writer George Orwell observed, "We may find in the long run that tinned food is a deadlier weapon than the machine gun." There is much to suggest that he may have been right.

Essentially, altered foods are what we call "processed"—that is foods which have been added to or changed by manufacturing. Most of our modern foods fall into this category. Consider these two examples:

White flour: Starts out as whole grain; ends up as white powder.

A grain of wheat contains a bran husk, a vitamin-rich "germ" and a starchy endosperm. Machine processing removes the fibrous and vitamin enriched parts and leaves the starchy center to be ground down to a fine, easily absorbed powder. The resulting product is so devoid of nutrients that since the 1940s, the government has mandated that various vitamins be added back—the reason flours are marked "enriched." Bleaching, additives, and preservatives may round out the package.

Margarine: Starts as vegetable oil; ends up as trans fat.

Arguably the most processed product in your market, margarine is made in factories, which pump hydrogen molecules into vegetable oil at high temperatures. This changes what was originally the flexible structure of the oil. It hardens and twists the framework so that it is essentially frozen in a new, artificial configuration—what is called a transfat. This allows the oil to stay hard so that it can be used as a spread. It also prevents the natural spoilage that would occur if the oil were left alone. Unfortunately trans-fats have turned out to be very harmful compounds. You will read more about this shortly.

Altered foods bear little resemblance to the simple products of our earth and have no precedent in the human diet. While not exactly plastic, they are certainly tampered with enough to be nutritionally questionable.

Why POWs Should Choose to Eat as Primarians

We have already talked about the fact that those who have been previously overweight (POWs) are different from those who have never been heavy (NOWs). In my work with POWs, I have observed time and again their extreme sensitivity to insulin promoting foods, in other words, S Foods.

POWs have two particular problems with these foods. First, they cause weight gain quickly. Second, they cause cravings, hunger and addiction. This has always been obvious in practice, but now we have emerging science to back up our observation. Work from Sweden, for example, has compared the effectiveness of a Paleolithic style diet (no grains) with the Mediterranean diet (heavy on whole grains) in subjects with Struggling Insulin Syndrome and heart disease. Experts proclaim the Mediterranean diet as "healthy." Yet these particular subjects had significantly greater decreases in weight, blood sugar, and insulin when they ate an ancient (grainless) diet. This early evidence would seem to confirm that those with a tendency towards Struggling Insulin Syndrome should restrict S Foods.

Remember that signs of Struggling Insulin Syndrome include some or all of the following: a history of belly fat, high blood pressure, elevated cholesterol or triglycerides, low good cholesterol, and a borderline or elevated blood sugar. While not all POWs have Struggling Insulin Syndrome, a very significant number do. Many more have a tendency to develop it in the future. In fact, I'll take it one step further. It is my belief that the majority of POWs will develop some degree of Struggling Insulin Syndrome if they continue to consume the modern American diet. Your best bet is to reduce the stress on your insulin-producing pancreas by eating Primarian.

The Quest for the Perfect Diet: Searching Here, There and Everywhere for Something That's Right in Front of Us

Thousands of papers and articles are written each year about the possible components of the perfect diet. Certain things are completely obvious. Study after study has concluded that there is great benefit to eating foods such as fruits and vegetables, nuts, fish, and poultry. In contrast, just as many studies document the harm of saturated fats, rapidly digested starches and simple sugars.

Imagine that we wanted to construct the perfect diet: one low in saturated fat and full of fruits and vegetables. Does that diet sound familiar? It should, because it fits the profile of the original, ancient diet.

Still not convinced? Let's look at a number of other current beliefs about the constituents of the perfect diet:

1. It should be low in salt.

You might be interested to know that ancients ate almost no salt. Today, 95 percent of men and 75 percent of women eat a diet that exceeds safe upper limits. Instead of eating about 1.5 grams of salt, we eat 6 grams or more.

Recently, the AMA issued a call for restaurants and food processors to decrease the salt in food. Excess salt is significantly linked to high blood pressure, an American killer. To underscore the seriousness of the AMA's effort Dr. Stephen Havas said, "The deaths attributable to excess sodium intake represent a huge toll—the equivalent of a jumbo jet with more than 400 adults crashing every day of the year, year after year." Do you need added salt? No.

Which diet gets salt right? The Primarian one.

2. It should be low in saturated fat.

Saturated fat raises the risk of heart disease. Major sources are cheese, butter, whole milk, fatty meat, and baked goods. The Primarian diet contains none of these foods and so vastly limits the risks associated with saturated fat consumption. Score another one for Primarian eating.

3. It should be high in omega-3 fatty acids.

There are two types of fats that you must get through diet as they cannot be manufactured in the body. These are the "essential" omega-3 and omega-6 fats. These fatty acids are involved in the body's ability to create inflammation (among other things). Omega-6 encourages inflammation and omega-3 calms it. We need both, in just the right ratio. Unfortunately, today's diet has ten times more omega-6 than omega-3. Why?

One of the major reasons is that omega-6 acids are prominently found in corn and other vegetable oils (safflower, soy, peanut, sunflower, sesame, and cottonseed). We use tremendous amounts of these oils in cooking and in packaged foods. Omega-3 acids, on the other hand, are found in less commonly consumed foods: cold water fish like tuna, salmon, mackerel, herring, and sardines and flax seed and nuts (macadamias and walnuts are especially good).

The excessive amount of omega-6 in our diet is a problem that makes us prone not only to inflammation but to abnormal blood clotting and heart arrhythmias. You probably won't be surprised to hear that all we need to do to restore the proper balance is to eat a Primarian diet. Ancient foods provided the perfect ratio.

4. It should be high in fiber.

Because of all the fruits, vegetables, and primary foods he consumed, ancient man's fiber intake was closer to 150 grams per day than our current 20 grams or less daily. Naturally, when you eat anciently, your fiber intake will soar.

5. It should be low in trans fats.

The food villain "du jour" is trans-fat, a compound that fully deserves its evil reputation. Trans-fats are particularly damaging to blood vessels. In fact, they appear to be worse for us than saturated fats. They not only raise levels of "bad" cholesterol (LDL) but lower levels of "good cholesterol" (HDL). In fact, Harvard's Nurse's Health Study found that women who ate an average of four teaspoons of stick margarine a day had 50 percent more heart disease than women who rarely ate margarine.

As early as 1994, Harvard professor Walter Willett indicted trans-fats as potentially responsible for 30,000 premature deaths per year, yet it wasn't until January 2006 that mandatory trans-fat food labeling appeared on products.

The safe amount of trans fat in your diet is zero. Remember that labels on foods that claim to have no trans fats can still conceal small amounts (up to half a gram). Always read food label ingredients. Foods that contain trans fats will have the words, "partially hydrogenated," "hydrogenated," or "vegetable shortening." If you see these words, do not eat what is in the package. Eating Primarian is the best way to eliminate trans fats. They do not appear significantly in the natural world.

6. It should be high in vitamins and minerals.

Potassium, magnesium, zinc, and other vitamins and minerals were much more plentiful when we ate anciently. Now, we take pills to boost their concentration in our diet. Most studies have shown that vitamins in pill form do not provide the same benefit as those contained in real foods.

Our current diet contains large loads of carbohydrate "filler," mostly starch and sugars that are devoid of the micronutrients we need. The Primarian diet with its load of fruits and vegetables is a vitamin and mineral powerhouse.

Have you gotten the point? The diet we're trying so hard to produce with all of our recommendations is very simply the one human beings always consumed.

It would be great if we could keep eating our modern diet and make small "tweaks" to correct deficiencies. But we've tried this and it doesn't work. Current recommendations, like "eat more fruits and vegetables" are based on the idea that adding "good" things to an unhealthful diet can counteract the "bad" parts. I don't believe this and our current state of health doesn't support it.

Why just add a few excellent foods to a mediocre diet? What if we ate entirely from an ancient menu? Could we achieve new levels of health?

The answer to this question can be found in years of observations made on ancient-eating cultures. Innumerable researchers have documented that people who eat primary diets do not develop "the modern diseases" that ravage many of us: vascular disease, diabetes, obesity, high blood pressure, and high cholesterol. While primitive peoples of the past often died young, their deaths resulted from accidents, infant mortality, and infection. Fossil records confirm that ancient peoples who lived into old age were free of our modern chronic illnesses.

Signs of Struggling Insulin Synrome: a history of belly fat, high blood pressure, elevated cholesterol or triglycerides, low good cholesterol, and a borderline or elevated blood sugar.

We can see this data replicated in the health of the few tribal peoples remaining today. These societies remain largely free from diseases of civilization. In Kenya, for example, two tribes of hunter-gatherers—the Masai and Kikuyu—have continued to exist into modernity. They were studied in 1931 when they were more populous and, although one tribe was meat-eating and the other vegetarian, neither appeared to suffer from Western disease.

More immediate evidence of the benefits of ancient diet comes from a dramatic study performed in Australia in 1982. Ten westernized Aborigines who suffered from Struggling Insulin Syndrome and diabetes agreed to return to the bush for seven weeks of a traditional hunter-gatherer diet. In this short period of time, their lipid levels and blood pressure fell and the level of omega-3 fats in their body tissues rose greatly. In addition, every one of their insulin abnormalities either improved markedly or returned to normal. This is direct and dramatic change indeed.

Until recently, Australian Aborigines lived free of modern diseases, maintaining low weights and eating a varied diet of meat, fish, and plant foods. Today, Aborigines who live a westernized life have rates of coronary disease that tragically exceed those of the general population. A similar decline in health has been seen time and again as ancient diets have given way to modern ones.

A completely ancient diet is often called "Paleolithic." My take on original diet, Primarian eating, is slightly modified from the more strict Paleolithic approach. I have tailored it to you, the weight maintainer. It is a bit less restrictive to allow maintainers to continue its use over long periods. For this reason it includes modest consumption of two new-comer foods: low fat dairy and non-starchy legumes. I suggest you use the name Primarian when you tell people how you eat. Explain the principles to those who ask. Like vegetarians, maintainers will benefit from having a named diet that easily defines their eating choice for others.

Why All of This Matters

Our modern diet leans heavily on Newcomer and altered foods while primary foods are largely ignored. In the last two chapters, we talked about the hormonal design of your body and discussed the fact that we humans have a rather fragile mechanism for processing S Foods (starch and sugar). Now we can see why we were designed this way. For most of our history S Foods were rare.

Newcomer foods changed everything by moving our diet heavily toward grain consumption. This may have had less impact when we ate sparingly, lived shorter lives and were heavily active, but as we moved into the altered food years, large loads of sugar were added to all that starch. Worse, the starches themselves were milled to become finer and easier to absorb. We were soon awash in blood sugar and insulin.

If you are a POW, someone who was once heavy, you have already proven that you gain weight easily when you eat the modern diet. You will remain highly sensitive to newcomer foods and altered foods because of the years of stress your insulin mechanism has already shouldered. Don't dare your body to restart the gain cycle with S Foods that tax insulin even more. This is a battle you can't win. It will lead to insulin overproduction, cravings, and the avid storage of fat. Just like the Aborigines who returned to the bush, you can return to a Primarian diet. Then the stress will be taken off insulin, levels will decline, and normal fat metabolism will resume.

To give yourself the best possible shot at successful maintenance, follow Primarian guidelines as completely as you possibly can for the first three months of maintenance, and 90 percent of the time thereafter as long as weight is maintained. (The 12 Tough Rules section will give you more guidance on this point.)

Food for Thought (Calorie-Free!)

It is my belief that no one, fat or thin, can healthily tolerate a diet they were not genetically built to eat. There is no doubt, though, that some people are more sensitive than others to eating grains and altered foods. As a POW (previously overweight), you fall into this camp. Your tendency to gain weight in the past proves that you are among the most sensitive to the deleterious effects of modern eating. But take heart; it also proves that you have a beautiful, pure, ancient physiology. Your genetic tendency to gain easily will not mutate, disappear, or suspend itself simply because you have lost weight. If anything, you have become more sensitive to these foods now that you are smaller. But you can disable the mechanism of weight gain by eating in harmony with what your genes expect. Trying to outwit biology is a losing proposition. Instead of fighting a losing battle, focus instead on experiencing yourself as a lovely, unchanged, primary soul while you honor your timeless heritage with every bite of food you consume.

Chapter Wrap

- Primarian foods are the original, simple foods of our planet. They include lean animal products, vegetables, fruits, eggs, fish, nuts, seeds, and berries.
- Our genetic makeup is designed to eat the foods that humans ate for millions of years.
- We are poorly designed to eat modern, altered foods.
- In addition to minimizing altered foods, POWs should also avoid grains and other Newcomer starches.

Chapter Six

Practical Ancient Eating

Tell me what you eat, and I will tell you what you are.
    —Jean-Anthelme Brillat-Savarin, *Physiologie Du Gout*

So now you know. Your guiding principle for maintenance eating is both simple and elegant: eat only what nature intends you to eat. In this chapter we will talk about the specifics of that food choice and the practical steps that will take you from modern eater to Primarian. Your new eating style will:

- Allow you to eat enough volume to feel satisfied.
- Provide you with optimum nutrition and excellent health.
- Prevent you from craving sweets and starches.
- Keep your hunger levels low.
- Keep weight where you want it.

What Primarians Eat

Primarians eat up-to-date versions of ancient foods—those which would have been available to hunter-gatherers in the wild. However, in order to make this eating style more flexible for you, I have also included some foods which are not strictly ancient but will work to give you more variety.

These are the foods that make up the Primarian menu:

Ancient:
    Lean meats
    Lean poultry
    Fish
    Other seafood
    Eggs
    Vegetables

Fruits
Berries
Nuts and seeds

Not ancient:
    Low-fat or non-fat dairy
    Selected oils
    Non-starchy legumes
    Occasional alcohol
    Acceptable treats

The newer foods I've included do not appear to cause weight gain or cravings when consumed reasonably. Adding them to your diet allows greater flexibility and permits an easier transition, but keep consumption of these foods modest. *Choose from the ancient foods list most frequently.*

Together, these two lists make up the Primarian Diet. You should select Primarian foods 90 to 100 percent of the time. This means that, with rare exception, you will build your meals from the foods listed above. *All other foods should be consumed very occasionally, mindfully, and in small amounts.*

Here is the Primarian Food List in greater detail:

Foods to eat

1. Lean meats:
    a. Choose any meat that is lean and has minimal visible fat.
    b. Lean red meat includes flank steak, sirloin, top round and eye round, leg of lamb and grass fed beef (see box below).
    c. Lean pork includes tenderloin and trimmed pork chops.
    d. Game meats include venison, bison, ostrich, and rabbit.

2. Poultry:
    a. Choose any type of poultry.
    b. Eat without skin most of the time. Note that white meat is leaner than dark.

3. Fish:
    a. Choose any type.
    b. Include cold water fish like salmon, mackerel, herring, sardines, and tuna, which contain beneficial omega-3 fats.

Grass-Fed Beef

In addition to eating what nature planned, it's a good idea to choose meat that comes from animals that are fed their ancient diet as well. One such choice is grass-fed beef. You can find this product at specialty grocers such as Whole Foods Market or order it online. Be sure to ask questions about the beef you buy as the quality varies. The appendix contains a list of questions for providers.

Why consider grass-fed meat? Cattle do not eat grain in their natural state, yet feedlots fatten them on exactly that—corn. This unnatural diet creates an overly acidic rumen (stomach) which allows bacteria to pass into the blood. In order to head off infection, large doses of antibiotics must be added to the daily ration. None of this is necessary when cattle are fed on pasture.

Corn and the addition of growth hormones speed up growth, allowing calves to reach full size within 14 to 16 months. Without such interventions, it would take a calf four or five years to grow to the same size. The resulting meat is modern, altered, and higher in fat and cholesterol than pasture-fed.

c. If you like canned fish, select the water packed variety.

4. Seafood:

a. Choose any type, including shrimp, scallops, mussels, crab, clams, oysters, lobster, octopus, eel, and squid.

5. Eggs:

a. If you do not have diabetes or high cholesterol, feel free to eat up to five to six eggs per week. For diabetics or those with cholesterol problems, choose egg whites as often as you like or mix two egg whites with a single egg yolk when cooking, a few times weekly.

b. You may also want to look for eggs that come from chickens fed with omega-3 fatty acids. This will increase your own omega-3 intake. These eggs are now available in most markets.

6. Vegetables:

a. Go heavy on the vegetables. Choose any vegetable except

potatoes, sweet potatoes, yams, and corn (note that corn is not a vegetable, it is a grain).

b. Be sure to include many dark leafy greens such as spinach, romaine lettuce, leaf lettuce, mustard and collard greens, chard, and kale.

c. Choose vegetables with many different colors, as the colors are markers of the nutrients within.

7. Fruits:

a. Eat any fresh fruit.

b. Watch the scale and limit consumption of very sweet tropical fruits like banana, pineapple, mango, and papaya.

c. Take care with dried fruit. It is fruit, but the drying process concentrates sugars. Many dried fruit products are also sweetened with high fructose corn syrup. It's OK to eat dried fruit, but look for an unsweetened version and watch the scale.

8. Berries:

a. Eat any type of berry.

9. Nuts and Seeds:

a. Eat any type of nut or seed.

b. Walnuts have particular benefit because of their high omega-3 content.

c. Eat nuts unsalted.

d. Watch the scale as nuts are calorie dense. The scale will tell you how many you can tolerate.

e. Avoid consumption of peanuts, which are actually part of the legume family and not a nut.

10. Non-caloric beverages:

a. Choose water, coffee, tea, diet sodas, and other diet drinks.

b. Many dieters feel that it's important to drink incessantly. Don't overdo it. Overzealous water drinking can actually dilute your blood causing a dangerous drop in sodium. These low levels have occurred in several of my patients after they drank large amounts of water while dieting. Primarian foods contain lots of fluids in the form of vegetable and fruit matter. Drink additionally only when you feel thirsty or if physical activity demands it.

11. Oils:
a. Limit cooking oils to olive, canola, and avocado oil. (When cooking with olive or avocado oils, try mixing them with canola oil to improve the balance of omega fats.)
b. To dress salads and vegetables, try a sprinkle of flaxseed or walnut oil. Do not cook with these two oils as they break down when heated. (Flaxseed oil is an excellent source of omega-3 fats.)
c. Use oils sparingly as they are calorie dense.
d. Do not use corn oil or other vegetable oils. While these oils are "polyunsaturated" (a type of fat we've come to think of as healthy), they actually contain a large percentage of omega-6 fats. Because so many packaged foods contain vegetable oil, we have been deluged with an unbalanced load of omega-6, which tends to promote inflammation. Confine your oils to the few recommended above.

12. Non-starchy legumes:
a. These are the beans that look more like vegetables and include string beans, snow peas, peas, and sugar snap peas.
b. Starchy beans (the kind that give you gas) and other legumes (lentils, peanuts, chickpeas, etc.) are not on the Primarian menu.

13. Non-fat and low-fat dairy products, as tolerated:
a. Non-fat and low-fat sour cream, cottage cheese, yogurt, milk, and cheese.
b. Be careful of added sugars in these products, especially in yogurts, fat-free ice creams, and puddings. (Check labels and look for lower carbohydrate counts. Avoid those sweetened with high fructose corn syrup.)
c. We do not need as much dairy as we think. If you choose to eat dairy, confine yourself to one or two servings a day.
d. If you are lactose intolerant, skip the dairy. Take a calcium supplement (about 1000-1500 mg/day) plus vitamin D (400-800 units/day).

14. Alcohol:

   a. Limit yourself to one drink daily, two maximum. Watch the scale.

   b. While many experts suggest that alcohol benefits health, this assumption is made in the context of the modern diet. Most ancient peoples were very healthy without the benefit of a daily drink. If you eat a Primarian diet, don't feel that you need to add alcohol.

   c. If you choose a mixed drink, use non-caloric mixers only. Alcohol contains 7 calories per gram weight, almost twice the calorie content of carbohydrate. Those calories add up quickly, especially when mixed with sodas, juices, and syrups. While a glass of wine has about 90 calories, a mixed drink can have as many as 700 or more.

A Double Whammy

In 2005, *Forbes* magazine published a list of the ten most fattening cocktails which included a Long Island Iced Tea (780 calories) a Piña Colada (644 calories), and a Margarita (740 calories). Since drinking tends to lower our inhibitions, alcohol also increases weight by making it easier for us to eat more.

In addition alcohol has another lesser known effect on the body. When we drink our bodies stop burning fat at the normal rate. Not only is alcohol caloric but it also slows down our own ability to use up the fat we would normally burn. Together this combination accelerates weight gain.

---

15. Acceptable treats:

   a. These are modern treats that are sweet and delicious but do not overly stimulate the appetite. Examples are low-fat pudding cups, low-fat sugar-free jello, low-fat frozen yogurt and ice cream products, and low-fat toppings. See Tough Rule 9 for more information on adding acceptable treats to the diet.

   b. There is room for one acceptable treat per day in the Primarian plan.

16. Helpful additions to the Primarian eating plan:

   a. Salad Dressing—Since there are a lot of vegetables and greens in the Primarian plan, most people want to know what salad dressings are acceptable.

i. Choose dressings which contain less than 20 calories per serving or make your own from the healthy oils above. Any vinegar is fine to use. You may want to try some of the No Calorie dressings (see resources) or salad sprays that are available.

ii. Always dip into dressing or drizzle small amounts on your salad. In restaurants, ask for salads with dressing on the side or, better yet, carry your own dressing packets in pocket or purse.

b. Mayonnaise—The soybean oil, which is combined with eggs in most commercial mayo is not one of our recommended oils. If you like mayonnaise, use just a touch. Diluting the mayonnaise with a small amount of water allows you to spread the flavor, yet use less. Light versions are less caloric.

c. Sugar substitutes—Use your favorite type for sweetening foods. Sucralose holds up to higher heats and is a better choice for cooking.

S Foods: Foods to Be Avoided

We could stop right here, because any foods other than the ones listed above should be eaten only occasionally and in small amounts. For POWs, though, it is particularly important that you diligently limit S Foods, so I want to describe these in more detail.

Limitation does not mean that you can never have an S Food again, but it does mean that you should avoid them most of the time and always approach them with caution. See Tough Rule 5 for more information.

Here is where I will ask you to be tough. I have found that elimination of S Foods most of the time is critical if you are to successfully maintain weight. Think of choosing an S Food as you used to think of choosing a hot fudge sundae—something you eat once in a great while and only after thinking about it first.

Stay away from (pass on these foods 90 percent of the time):

Grain—This includes whole grains (wheat, rye, oats, barley, —all grains).

Corn—Remember, it's a grain and not a vegetable. This includes popcorn.

Cereals—All cereals, including oatmeal and whole grain cereals, "healthy" granolas, etc....

Products made from flour—Breads, muffins, bagels, pancakes, pizza crust, tortillas, flat breads, pita, crackers, noodles, etc., whether "whole grain" or not.

Rice—All types, including brown and wild rice.

Potatoes—White, sweet, and yams.

Sugar—All added sugar including high fructose corn syrup and other sugar-based sweeteners, such as maple syrup and molasses.

Honey.

Juices (always choose whole fruit instead).

Sweets—Candy, cake, cookies, doughnuts, and regular ice creams.

Pasta—All types including whole grain pasta.

Sweetened drinks—Regular sodas, non-diet iced teas, and fruit drinks, etc. Be sure to check labels for the presence of sugars. Drink only if calorie count is zero.

There are a number of other foods that don't appear on the Primarian list and should be completely avoided or eaten only now and then. Some are worthy of comment.

- **Anything with trans fats:** Even if the label says a product contains zero grams, you can detect the presence of non-reportable amounts by looking for the words "hydrogenated" or "partially hydrogenated" in the ingredient list. Avoid completely.

- **Bacon, sausage, hot dogs, deli meats:** Although these are meats, they are highly processed, fatty, contain a higher percentage of bad fats, and are excessively salted. Some also are preserved with nitrites, a potentially dangerous additive. Consider low-salt alternatives or lean versions. Eat only occasionally.

- **Fried foods:** Regardless of the type of oil used, frying elevates the calories of food. Heating oils to a high temperature can also create harmful compounds. Eat rarely.

- **Things with lots of salt:** Choose low salt alternatives. Do not add salt to your food. Cook with minimal amounts and only if needed for flavoring.
- **Things in packages with long lists of unpronounceable ingredients:** Many of these processed foods contain S Food elements like corn, flour, wheat, or potatoes. Stick to foods with names you understand.
- **Full-fat dairy:** Cheese, milk, butter, cream, whipped cream, sour cream, ice cream, and other dairy products that are not reduced in fat contain high levels of saturated fat, the type of fat that raises cholesterol levels and has been implicated in vessel disease. Remember to choose non-fat or low-fat dairy.
- **"Heart Healthy" margarines:** The jury is out. They are still processed, have additives and are far from natural. Better to get out of the "spread" habit.
- **Starchy Beans:** You can think of these as the beans that give you "gas"—kidney beans, pinto beans, white and black beans, chickpeas, lentils, soybeans, etc. Beans are not Primarian foods and can promote weight gain because of their starchiness. On the other hand, most people have trouble eating too many of them and that limits their consumption. If you do eat beans, have a small amount and use occasionally to add some "heft" to a meal.
- **Condiments:** Ketchup, mustard, steak sauces, relishes, and chutneys can contain high amounts of sugars and salt. (Check labels for the presence of sugar or high fructose corn syrup.) You are better off using fresh fruit and vegetable salsas to accompany meals, but if you do prefer standard condiments, use just a little.

Making Your Primarian Plan Work
Step One: Treat your primarian diet as a "Diet of Conviction"

Perhaps you have noticed that people have no problem being judgmental about the eating habits of maintainers. My Maintenance Juniors routinely report being barraged by verbal digs:

"That diet is unhealthy."

"You're not having the bread? That's crazy!"

"You're not eating enough."

Clearly, it is socially acceptable to criticize the way post-dieters eat. On the other hand, it is considered in completely poor taste to disparage those eating a diet of conviction. By this, I mean an eating style that carries a name and is tied to a belief.

Some diets of conviction are: vegan, vegetarian, kosher, gluten-free, and CRON diets. Not a soul would suggest that a vegetarian stop the foolishness and order meat or that a Kosher person try a pork chop. People understand that these eating styles are based on personal, health, or religious beliefs. It is politically correct to respect them.

Always remember that your maintenance diet is very definitely a diet of conviction too. It is based on your desire for permanent health and your belief about how best to achieve it. It deserves respect. This is the reason I suggest that you use the word Primarian to identify your eating plan. It gives it a name and form. Explain the rules of Primarian eating if asked, and always say that you adhere to this diet for medical or philosophic reasons.

Here are a few simple ways to identify your diet:

- "Sorry, I can't have that. I'm a Primarian."
- "I follow a Primarian diet. It means I eat only ancient foods."
- "I'm a Primarian. It's a diet based on eating what you can hunt, gather, pick, or fish. I need to eat this way to control my (select one: diabetes, high blood pressure, cholesterol, heart disease, obesity)."

Step Two: Make it simple

Get rid of the endless concerns about proper percentages of carbohydrates and proteins, ratios of omega-3 to omega-6 acids, and grams of saturated versus unsaturated fats. In all my years of counseling people about weight, I have yet to meet anyone who followed a diet based on numbers or percents. While counting nutrients is of interest to the food scientist, it is not particularly helpful (at least on a daily basis) to the average person trying to construct a healthy diet.

The rules of your Primarian diet are easy to follow. By making the choice to eat anciently, you will automatically provide yourself with the right percentage of nutrients. When confronted with a food, ask yourself whether it could have been eaten by someone living in the wild. If the answer is no, don't eat it. If the answer is yes, go ahead and enjoy. Mix plenty of plant foods with your meat, fish, and poultry choices. The portions that you choose will be dictated by the scale. (Learn more about this in Section Two.)

Step Three: Eat via plate pattern

It's easy to know how to eat if you know what every plate should look like. When you fill a major meal plate, automatically envision the following pattern and place your foods accordingly:

- **One quarter of your plate: Lean animal foods**

Meat, poultry, fish, eggs, or low-fat dairy. Cheeses should be low-fat and used only as a sprinkle. Don't overdo the dairy. You will get plenty of calcium in your other foods and there are some potential concerns about dairy products. If calcium remains a worry, take a calcium supplement.

- **Three quarters of your plate: Plant foods**

Select unlimited amounts of fruits and vegetables and choose a wide variety of colors. Try to vary the types of plant foods you eat in order to get a good array. Although our American habit is to eat vegetables with a meal and fruit as a snack, there is no reason to ban fruits from the dinner plate. Try mixing slices of pear or apple with salad greens, or devote an entire corner to mixed fruits. Don't

Primarians eat up-to-date versions of ancient foods—those which would have been available to hunter-gatherers in the wild.

forget berries such as blueberries and strawberries which are high in antioxidant compounds. Antioxidants prevent and repair cell damage.

Include unsalted nuts and seeds if you enjoy them and sprinkle them right on your plate. Walnuts are especially good because of their high omega-3 content, but all nuts are fine. Remember, though, that nuts are caloric. Watch the scale and cut back if they are causing weight gain. For an additional boost to healthful omega-3 fats, add one to two tablespoons of ground flax seeds to your plate (buy whole seeds in a health food store and grind in coffee grinder daily). Ground flax can also be used to top yogurt, fruit, or salads.

- **Large salad on the side**

Dark leafy greens are particularly beneficial to health, so be sure to include foods like romaine lettuce, kale, chard, and spinach.

Many bagged salad mixes now contain dark greens, which will allow you to obtain them easily.

Giving Up the Gong

The Primarian way of life asks you to give up "Thrill Eating" (you know, the huge pile of mashed potatoes just for fun). It also asks you to give up "Gong Foods." These are the modern S Foods whose flavors are so potent that they explode in your mouth and remind you of that carnival game: the one in which you swing the hammer hard enough to get the bell to ring. Yes, it's goodbye to the gong. But here's why it's well worth it:

- Eating Primarian, you will quickly find a new balance, free of cravings and out from under the control of food.
- You'll be able to wake up in the morning without being angry at yourself and you'll be able to wear the same clothes you wore the day before.
- You will be uplifted by the knowledge that everything you eat is enhancing your body and nothing is harming it.
- You will experience the feeling of food as an ally, not a master.

Time to hunt and gather!

Chapter Wrap

- Your Primarian diet is based on lean animal products, fish, eggs, fruits, vegetables, low-fat dairy, nuts, and seeds.
- A good guideline for major meals is a three-quarter plate of vegetables, fruits, nuts, berries, and seeds and a one-quarter plate of animal protein. Add a salad on the side.
- Don't count or measure.
- Seek the leanest animal products and the lowest fat dairy.
- Look for meat and poultry that is raised on its naturally intended diet.
- Use low-fat dairy for variety, but do so sparingly.
- Be very tough about avoiding S Foods.
- Treat your diet as a diet of conviction and honor its importance by following it consistently, and by explaining it and defending it to others.

Chapter Seven

The S Foods or
That's Not Spaghetti in Your Blood

Type 2 diabetes is engulfing India, swallowing up the legs and jewels of those comfortable enough to put on weight in a country better known for famine. Here, juxtaposed alongside the stick-thin poverty, the malaria and the AIDS, the number of diabetics now totals around 35 million, and counting.
—*The New York Times*, September 13, 2006

We have already talked about the most profound of the many differences between our ancient Primarian diet and the one we eat today—the recent addition of huge amounts of sugars and starches to our food supply. The world's health is paying. In India, thousands of people are treated in "sugar hospitals," in China diabetes rates are soaring, and here in the U.S., the disease is devouring New York City. Since S Foods have become the dietary giants of the modern world, I have given them a chapter of their own.

In Chapter Three, we talked about the fact that starch equals sugar. As you know, the stomach and intestines quickly disassemble starches. Their basic sugar "blocks" are what pass into the bloodstream. If I obtain a blood test from you after you've eaten a bowl of pasta, I will find sugar—not spaghetti or starch molecules—in your blood.

Are Some S Foods Better than Others?

This is an interesting question. Many diet experts advocate a scale called the "glycemic index" to separate bad S Foods from better ones. Glycemic index is simply a measure of how quickly your body turns S Foods into blood sugar. Theoretically, S Foods that are released more slowly into the blood create fewer insulin problems. Newcomer foods such as whole grains, cereals, and beans contain fiber, and this fiber acts like a net, which traps sugar molecules so that they enter the blood more slowly. The question is, does this knowledge benefit you, the person who has a tendency to gain weight easily?

Here is my opinion. I personally don't find the use of glycemic index very helpful for Maintenance Juniors. Why not?

Because of their high rate of struggling insulin problems, POWs appear to be highly sensitive to all foods that turn into sugars. These foods tend to "addict" them as well. In my experience, it doesn't seem to matter if the sugars are released more slowly or not.

Many POWs notice that they gain weight when they reintroduce grains and products like whole wheat breads and pastas to their diet. This occurs even though these foods supposedly have a better glycemic index than other carbohydrates.

Using glycemic index means consulting lists and memorizing values. As I have said before, diet plans that rely on counting or memorization don't work very well long term.

Apart from my own opinion, two major research studies recently cast doubt on the usefulness of glycemic index; each appeared in the *American Journal of Clinical Nutrition*. The first study examined whether type 2 diabetics had better blood sugars if they ate a low glycemic index diet. They didn't. The second looked at whether eating low glycemic index foods could prevent diabetes from getting started in the first place. In both cases, consuming low glycemic index foods was ineffective. Whether these negative results occurred because glycemic index doesn't work in practice or because people found it too cumbersome to use, the end result was the same.

Rather than trying to separate good S Foods from bad, I recommend a marked decrease in intake of all S Foods. I advocate that you begin with a three month period of complete S Food avoidance. After this, if you attempt to add back small controlled amounts of S Foods, less altered forms (like whole grains), are clearly preferable to modern sweets. Even so, you should only experiment with these food types if they do not stimulate cravings and if the scale stays stable. My hope is that you will be so happy with your new life and health that you won't be particularly interested in experimenting with many S Foods. Experimentation often leads to maintenance disaster because, whatever its source, we can't seem to say no to food that is starchy or sweet.

Our Super Sweet World

How did sugars come to so dominate our diet? You may think of table sugar as an ancient food, but it's actually surprisingly modern. While natural honey has always been around, sugar from the sugar cane plant actually made its first appearance in Western Europe as late as the 11th century (around the time of the Crusades). Prior to this, sugar cane had been known in Persia and in India around 500 BC. This puts the introduction of sugar into the human diet at a mere 2,500 years ago.

Major world upheavals, including the initiation and sustenance of the Caribbean slave trade, have occurred because of sugar. Taxes have been levied, battles fought, untold fortunes have been made from its production. These facts should tell you something about the power of sugar and the degree to which humans crave sweetness. Yet, strangely, our bodies don't require added sugars. We lived largely without them for millions of years.

As late as 1750, sugar was still a luxury product in England, dubbed "white gold." At around this time, however, a new source appeared on the scene: the sugar beet. Even with this new means of production, sugar remained too expensive for most people until the latter part of the 19th century. Once prices came down and the average man could sweeten his foods, he did so with a vengeance. Someone living in the early 1800s ate about fifteen pounds of sugar a year. Fast forward to today. We each eat about 150 pounds of the stuff every year. It is worth noting that this figure does not include the additional load of blood sugar that comes from the starches we eat. The huge sugar load we ingest has no precedent in our past experience as a species.

First honey, then cane, then the sugar beet—sugar sources have changed with time. They did so again recently. During the 1970s, scientists found yet another way to produce sugar, one that was cheap and highly available. They found that starch from corn (starch equals sugar— remember?) could be treated and transformed into a sweet syrup called high fructose corn syrup (HFCS). Because the government had begun paying farmers to grow corn, there was a lot of it around. The excess meant that high fructose corn syrup could be produced cheaply, enabling it to be added in large amounts to many processed foods. As of 2005, a food manufacturer wanting to sweeten a product would have to pay 24 cents for a pound of beet-derived sugar, but just 13 cents for the same amount of HFCS.

The addition of HFCS, actually a blend of 55 percent fructose and 45 percent glucose, seems to have fueled our craving for ever more sweetness. It began to appear in a startling number of packaged foods and beverages.

From the 1920s to the 1960s, the average American steadily ate around 120 pounds of sugars each year. After the introduction of HFCS in the 1970s, however, this amount began climbing. By 2004, we were packing away 150 pounds per person per year as was mentioned earlier. Virtually all of this increase came from corn-based sweeteners. During the same time period, the amount of overweight and obesity in our country soared to record highs.

Did HFCS directly contribute to the obesity epidemic because it is uniquely fattening in some way? The jury is still out, but there is reason to wonder. The body processes fructose differently from other simple sugars. Unlike glucose, fructose proceeds directly to the liver rather than spending time in the bloodstream. Research from a number of labs suggests that the liver responds to this fructose load by making it into fat. Fructose may also cause worsening of Struggling Insulin Syndrome.

The next time you visit your supermarket, make a point to check packages, bottles, and cans for the presence of this ubiquitous additive. POWs should avoid it, just as they should avoid other added sugars.

Our Way-Too-Starchy World

As opposed to sugars, starches have a longer history in our diet. They made their first significant appearance during the Newcomer period, about 10,000 years ago. Prior to that time, humans ate small amounts of wild grain material and a few other starches contained in fibrous roots and tubers. These plants were nothing like the enormous potatoes or tall grains we cultivate today. During the Newcomer period, when farming began, wheat and barley were produced by cultivating the seeds of smaller wild grains. The production of rice and millet came slightly later. These were eaten as whole grains consumed with all their parts: endosperm, germ, and bran.

Records from around 350 BC document the early beginnings of making fine whitened flour from these whole grains. To do this, the starchy endosperm was separated from the grain's germ and husk—a rudimentary form of processing. So we can date the entry of processed grains into our diet at approximately 2,500 years ago.

The Greeks and Romans first introduced the idea that white flour was food for the elite. Slaves and other poor members of society were fed whole grain bread called panis sordidis (dirty bread). Despite the fact that pure white flours were sought after, grains continued to be ground mostly by mill stones until the late 1800s.

Things changed when the first modern milling machinery appeared. New industrial techniques allowed grains to be separated and pulverized into ever finer particles, creating the fine white flours that consumers preferred. While this flour looked lovely and made a light loaf, its pure appearance was achieved by ridding it of the nutrition-packed germ and bran. So devoid of nutrients was this final flour that, in 1941, the U.S. government mandated artificial "enrichment" of flour with niacin, riboflavin, thiamine, folic acid, and iron. According to General Mills' informational web site, this was done "as the result of diet studies in 1940 which showed that millions of Americans were suffering from inadequate diets."

Crushing, mashing, pulverizing, and otherwise smashing carbohydrates makes their sugars more available. Many of the products labeled "whole grain" on our shelves may have the germ and bran left in, but they are made from flours that have been very finely ground. Whole grain pastas, for example, are clearly not made from crunchy, hard pieces of grain. The same can be said for most cereals. Many breads claim to be "whole grain" but many have deceptively little whole grain included. For this and other reasons, I suggest that POWs treat grain products as if they were sugars. Those that came before us lived well without grain in their diet. Assuming that you are eating a highly healthful Primarian diet full of fruits, vegetables and lean protein, your body will not miss grains and the products made from them.

Are the S Foods Addictive? I Vote Yes

What is a drug? It is a chemical substance that affects the processes of the mind or the body. Drugs appear to be inert, but when ingested—they cause specific changes to occur. By this definition, food is a kind of drug. The mistake that most dieters make is in assuming that food is harmless, simple, and controllable. Food is none of these. Food is exactly like any other drug, a chemical substance which creates a cascade of effects when it is ingested. This chain reaction resonates in every cell of your body.

All drugs are not the same, and neither are all foods. An aspirin is a drug, but it has far different effects than a narcotic. I have yet to meet a patient who has told me that he or she is addicted to apples, salmon, or spinach. On the other hand, it is rare to meet a patient who does not use the language of addiction when describing his or her relationship to chocolate, cookies, pasta, or bread. Why is this? Different foods have different effects.

Why can't we stop eating S Foods? Because they are particularly drug-like. Recently, the FDA denied approval for Rimonabant, a weight loss drug currently used in Europe. This compound decreases appetite by blocking the same areas of the brain that are stimulated by marijuana. Most people know that pot smoking causes people to get hungry, a phenomenon known as "the munchies." It turns out that blocking these drug centers turns off appetite. This fact reinforces the fact that foods and drugs work similarly, even in the same brain areas. Unfortunately, in the case Rimonabant, blocking these pleasure areas caused an unacceptable incidence of depression, triggering the FDA's denial.

Researchers at Princeton University have shown that rats fed high levels of sugars will develop symptoms that look identical to drug withdrawal when sugar is discontinued. According these researchers, certain brain areas can be stimulated by both sweet foods and drugs, leading to similar types of "abuse and addiction."

But I don't have to tell you any of this. As a POW, you are only too aware of the addictive nature of your trigger foods.

> *Food is exactly like any other drug, a chemical substance which creates a cascade of effects when it is ingested.*

The key to beating S Foods is for you to exert the control by opting out of the drug. No drug, no power. If S Foods and drugs are comparable, we would be wise to take a page from addiction treatment. Stay clean of the substance that is causing your problem.

You can do this initially by committing to three perfect months of maintenance. After this, shoot for eating a diet devoid of S Foods 90 percent of the time. When and if you do eat S Foods, be extremely cautious. Once these foods begin to crawl back into your plan, they have an insidious way of taking over almost without your knowing it. I call this "Food Creep." Again, as a past dieter, I don't have to define food creep for you. You already know all about it.

You will need to be intensely vigilant, but if you continue to follow a Primarian plan, you will find that control actually becomes second nature in time. Your daily diet just becomes something that you do, and more important, something that you prefer to do.

Is a Calorie a Calorie? I Vote No

One of the most persistent debates in the weight loss world is whether a calorie of Snickers bar is the same as a calorie of broccoli. Many diets are built around the premise that you will lose weight eating 1,000 calories no matter whether they come from cheesecake or chicken breast. While it is clearly true that eating tiny amounts of any form of food will cause weight loss, observation tells us that foods are not equal.

We must stop looking at calories as the only way to define foods. The body response needed to utilize proteins is completely distinct from that which processes sugars. That alone makes these two forms of calories different. More important, there are two parts to any food equation: the nature of the food and the nature of the person who is eating that food. Scientists measure the energy (in calories) of a food by burning it in a machine called a calorimeter. One calorimeter is just like the next. But put that food into a human being and all bets are off. One human is not like the next and humans are not simple machines.

If someone overproduces insulin, his response to a sugar calorie will be quite different than that of a person with normal insulin function. Insulin fluxes stimulate intensely hungry feelings, for example. Thus, protein calories (which do not provoke large insulin releases) create much less hunger in such a person than sugar calories (which do). Yes, the calories may be the same, but calories only describe one property of food: the energy. Calories tell us nothing about the complicated body processes that each food stimulates.

Yet another reason a calorie is not a calorie involves the relative value of foods. A calorie of oak leaves is equal to a calorie of spinach, but only one can be eaten by a human being. A calorie of table sugar is equal to a calorie of blueberries, but one is completely devoid of vitamins, minerals, and phytonutrients while the other is a nutritional power house. In short, a calorie is very definitely not a calorie. Your choice of food remains important and affects the way your body uses energy. While the calories in food still have some significance, maintenance is much more about the types of calories you choose and those you choose to avoid.

Won't I Be Lacking Important Nutrition if I Cut Out Grains?

Not if you substitute healthy fruits, vegetables, and lean animal proteins for the foods you've eliminated. In 2002, Dr. Loren Cordain at Colorado State University analyzed a contemporary form of an ancient diet so that he could calculate its nutritional value. The diet had no grains, modern sugars, legumes, or processed starches. Unlike our Primarian plan, it also lacked dairy. Foods in the plan were limited to

	Total	% RDA
Vitamin A (RE)	6386	798
Vitamin B1 (mg)	3.4	309
Vitamin B2 (mg)	4.2	355
Vitamin B3 (mg)	60	428
Vitamin B6 (mg)	6.7	515
Folate (µg)	891	223
Vitamin B12 (µg)	17.6	733
Vitamin C (mg)	748	1247
Vitamin E (IU)	19.5	244
Calcium (mg)	691	69
Phosphorus (mg)	2546	364
Magnesium (mg)	643	207
Iron (mg)	24.3	162
Zinc (mg)	27.4	228

Trace nutrients in a modern diet based on Paleolithic food groups for females (25 years old, 2,200 kcal daily energy intake). Courtesy of Loren Cordain, Ph.D.

fruits, vegetables, fish, poultry, meat, nuts, and seeds. The aim was to find out if such a diet provided enough nutrients to be healthy.

Analysis showed that not only was this diet healthy, it actually exceeded recommended daily allowances for nearly every nutrient including vitamins A, C, and E; the B vitamin group; folate; magnesium; phosphate; and zinc. The only nutrients which fell below current daily requirements were calcium and vitamin D, but remember that the purely ancient diet excludes dairy, which is permitted in your Primarian plan (see Table). If you don't like or tolerate dairy, you can supplement your plan with a calcium supplement which includes vitamin D.

Your diet can be supremely healthy without grains, starches, or added sugars. Don't be afraid to try it.

Does the Primarian Plan Work Simply Because You Eat Less?

Good question. If you eliminate all breads, pastas, grains, and sweets, you cut out a major source of calories. Naturally, you'd expect this to result in better control of weight. Why not cut out something else and leave those delicious S Foods intact?

Once these S Foods begin to crawl back into your plan, they have an insidious way of taking over almost without your knowing it.

While Primarian eating may ultimately result in fewer calories, its uniqueness lies in the fact that it allows you to feel quite content with consuming less. Here are the reasons that Primarian choices work best for the POW:

- Because of its low demands on insulin, the Primarian menu is one of the only eating plans that keeps POWs from being continually hungry. This is vital for maintainers.
- Food "addicts" often complain that they can't control what they eat because, unlike those who have other addictions, they can't stop eating entirely. While that is true, they can completely eliminate S Foods without any nutritional consequences. Eliminating these foods will noticably cut their cravings.
- Once S Foods are removed, there is a lot of room left for large amounts of extremely healthy foods.

- The Primarian diet completely removes calories that carry no nutritional punch—what are called "empty calories." Every bite is healthy.

Chapter Wrap

- S Foods are sugars and starches. Both result in sugar in the blood.
- S Foods are Newcomers to the human diet and are not essential for health, so long as the rest of the diet is full of nutrients.
- In POWs, S Foods trigger hunger and weight gain.
- S Foods have addictive qualities.
- Take S Foods out of your diet for successful long-term maintenance.

Chapter Eight

Understanding Your New Metabolism

It may seem logical to think that significant weight gain or being overweight is related to a low metabolism.... In reality, it's very uncommon for excess weight to be related to a low metabolism.
—Mayo Clinic Website (mayoclinic.com)

A particularly confusing topic for many dieters is the subject of metabolism. Let's discuss what metabolism really means and, more importantly, what effect your recent weight loss has had on your metabolic rate.

When I ask my patients to tell me what they know about metabolism they often say:

"Thin people have fast metabolisms."
"I don't know exactly what metabolism is, but mine is very slow."
"I hope that when I lose weight, my metabolism will improve."

In other words, while most overweight people are not too sure about the definition, they remain pretty certain that their own metabolism is sub-standard.

Metabolism: What Is It?

Metabolism is a measure of all of the business conducted by your body. We assign a value to it by figuring out how many calories you burn in a day.

Here are the major ways that your body burns calories (uses energy):

Organ and cell work

Your body factory powers a major pump (your heart), busy transportation systems (your blood vessels, nerves, and digestive systems), and lots of other moving parts. All of your organs must burn calories in order to keep working. Some examples of interior jobs that require fuel are:

- Breathing
- Detoxification of materials
- Cellular work
- Brain tasks
- Waste removal

This internal work is distinct from any moving around that you do. These calories are burned even if you are resting or sleeping. We call these calories your "resting metabolic rate"—how much your body burns when it's not active.

Muscle work

Obviously, working your body hard by asking it to run, lift, sweat and strain burns calories. But your body also burns a significant number of calories in minor physical activities. Walking from place to place, standing up, even jiggling your leg while you're sitting in a chair—these all burn calories.

Food digestion work

The process of eating and burning up food also takes energy. Some people burn more calories when digesting than others. This part of metabolism is called the "thermic effect of food." It is not measured by metabolic testing but usually represents a small number of calories.

Measures of metabolism can be done with complicated machinery or, more recently, with hand-held devices available in some doctors' offices. After breathing into these small machines for a few minutes, your resting metabolic rate can be calculated. Since resting metabolism doesn't tell us anything about muscle work, the tester will ask you how much exercise you do and add a factor based on your activity level to calculate your total daily metabolic rate.

What Factors Can Affect Your Metabolism?

Once again, metabolism is simply the calories, or energy, you use. Some factors can alter this usage. If your thyroid is overactive, for example, the excessive thyroid hormone drives your heart to beat faster and pushes other body processes to move at a quicker speed. Like stepping on the gas pedal this acceleration causes the burning of more fuel. If more energy is burned, that means metabolic rate is higher. Some medicines that you take may affect power output as well. Amphetamines are called "speed" because they speed up body work and cause more calorie burning. Other medicines, like the blood pressure medications called "beta blockers," may slow you down. In addition, there are a number of common medicines that are associated with weight gain, possibly because of metabolic effects.

Common Medications that Cause Weight Gain:

Psychiatric Drugs: SSRIs, tricyclics, MAOIs, phenothiazines
Mood Stabilizing Drugs: Lithium, sodium valproate
Anticonvulsants: Gabapentin, valproic acid, carbamazepine
Antipsychotics: Including olanzapine, clozapine, and risperidone
Migraine Preventatives: Valproic acid, gabapentin, tricyclics, SSRIs, beta blockers
Diabetes Drugs: Insulin, sulfonylureas, thiazolidinediones
Others: Estrogen, progesterone, steroids, antihistamines, alpha and beta blocker blood pressure medicines

---

If you are taking medications, check with your physician about those that might be associated with weight gain. Alternatives are often available.

Let's assume, though, that your thyroid is in order and you are not on weight-altering medication. Given this, there are a number of things we can say about metabolism.

Big burns more

Here's a question: which burns more fuel—a tractor trailer or an economy car? Simple, right? The truck is a gas guzzler compared to the tiny vehicle. Big burns more. This is true for people as well. A large, overweight person burns substantially more calories per day than a small person. Whether at rest or on the move, it takes more energy to run a bigger vehicle. Heavy people also have developed larger stores of muscle to support their weight. Muscle is a calorie burning tissue. Calories burned = metabolism. Therefore, who has the higher metabolic rate—a skinny person or an obese person? This answer often surprises people: it's the obese person.

Youth burns more/age burns less

Which vehicle burns more fuel: A car with a souped up engine or a no-frills model? Again, simple logic tells us that the more complicated engine burns more. Younger people have more calorie-burning muscle on their bodies. They are more "souped up" than their older. counterparts. A consequence of aging is the replacement of muscle by fatty tissue, tissue which does not burn calories. The result? As we age, we burn fewer calories and thus have slower metabolisms.

Men and muscles burn more

Larger and more muscular people burn more calories. This translates into a difference between men and women. Because men have more muscle mass and are larger, their metabolisms are faster than those of women. In other words, their bodies burn more calories per day.

Here's what you just learned. Your metabolism is mostly a function of three things: your size, your age, and your sex. Pretty simple and straightforward. Yet many people who have had weight issues secretly believe that there is "something wrong" with their own metabolism. Chances are you might believe the same thing about yourself. Could you be right?

Most of Us Have Normal Metabolisms for Our Size

While it is always possible that you could be one of the "metabolically challenged," the chances are—that in terms of calories burned—you are within the normal range. For many years scientists and physicians have used mathematical equations to predict the number of calories people burn each day: their metabolic rate. Machines that directly measure metabolism can now check if these predictions are correct. Someone with an abnormally slow metabolism, for example, would have a breathing test that shows far fewer calories burned than an equation would have predicted.

In practice, though, the best of these equations work pretty well to accurately predict what the real-life test will show. This means that most people have metabolisms that fall within the normal range for their size, age, and sex. Since "big burns more," this means that overweight patients generally measure out to have generous metabolic rates—not abnormally slow ones. This also means, that when you were heavier and had larger calorie needs, you were probably eating a lot of calories to keep up.

If you are still worried about an abnormal metabolism, have a resting metabolic rate test performed. Chances are you will discover it is just fine. Even should you be the rare metabolically challenged individual, metabolism is not destiny. If the world was filled with lean people in a past time, you can be assured that your problem has come not from your genes or your metabolic rate, but from your body's interaction with a food environment it was never meant to encounter.

Wait for several months after your weight loss diet is over before testing metabolic rate. This allows your metabolic rate, which may have been somewhat suppressed by dieting, to come back to normal.

Metabolism vs. Metabolic Syndrome

Just a reminder. Metabolic Syndrome and metabolism are not the same thing. Remember that Metabolic Syndrome, or Struggling Insulin Syndrome, is a complex of conditions that accompanies visceral fat. It has nothing to do with metabolic rate or to the type of metabolism we are discussing in this chapter (one of the reasons that I think the name is confusing).

You may have Metabolic Syndrome and still have a perfectly normal metabolism.

How Did Your Weight Loss Affect Your Metabolism?

So it's settled. Before your weight loss, you were probably burning an appropriate amount of calories for your size, age, and weight. Now let's use our understanding of metabolism to talk about you in your new incarnation as a Maintenance Junior. What has happened to your metabolism, or ability to burn calories, as a result of your weight loss?

Many people have heard that diets are a bad idea because they cause metabolism to be suppressed. While it's true that your body responds to restriction of calories by temporarily turning down its calorie burn (and the topic remains controversial) there is a lot of evidence that says that metabolism returns to normal once the diet over.

The National Weight Control Registry reports that they do not find any "metabolic impairment" in their weight maintainers and that those they examined did not show a metabolic rate that was lower than predicted for their new size. The last part of this sentence is important, because while the process of dieting does not permanently affect your metabolism, there is something else that does: your smaller body.

Remember the tractor trailer and the economy car? Which were you at the beginning of your diet and which are you now? As you now know, small burns less. Therefore you now have a metabolic rate which is lower than where you started. This is incredibly annoying, but it is to be expected. It is predicted by those pesky rules of metabolism.

There are a couple of other problems that loom for our metabolism as well. The first is our unfortunate tendency to get older every day. No matter what we do, our metabolic burn is inevitably going to slow down in time (age burns less). Second, significant amounts of weight loss always involve the loss of some muscle along with fat. You undoubtedly have less muscle now than you did when you began your diet. Since muscle burns calories, (muscles burn more) this puts you at a bit of a disadvantage too.

Your metabolism is mostly a function of three things: your size, your age, and your sex.

Most POWs do not take their new, smaller body size into account after a diet. They generally don't realize that this new body is going to need lots fewer calories to run. While most post-dieters try to eat healthier, they don't significantly reduce calories when compared to what they ate before. This is one of the major reasons they regain weight. Calories are still important in weight maintenance.

Successful maintenance requires a fully rebuilt diet that relies on significantly fewer calories than you ate when you were heavy. Exercise can really help now. If you would prefer to eat a bit more, you can do so by burning off some of what you eat with additional, vigorous activity.

Exercise may benefit metabolism as well. One study which looked at maintainers eighteen to forty months after dieting showed that those who exercised had normal metabolic rates for size, whereas those who were sedentary had slower than predicted rates. If you want to be assured of a nice, active metabolic rate—exercise. Be sure to include some muscle building activity to maintain a good store of metabolically active muscle tissue.

It seems almost unfair that your new body is so self-sufficient. It just doesn't need a lot of food to run. But rejoice! You have simply returned your physiology to its normal state of affairs. Healthy, efficient bodies work really well on small amounts of high quality food. Your new body is now functioning perfectly!

Patients on weight loss diets (you may have experienced this) often comment that they feel unusually well when they are eating a minimal amount of food. When they fall off the wagon and are plopped back into the food flood, they are bothered by more than just guilty conscience. They actually feel physically uncomfortable for a time. So eat "scarcely." Don't be afraid of the fact that your body needs less now. Respect its wishes. If you stay away from hunger stimulating S Foods, you will be surprised at how readily you learn to eat less.

How much food is appropriate for your new metabolism? It will take a bit of experimenting to find out. The entire trick is to eat as much Primarian food as you can without exceeding what I call your "Scream Weight." You alone will be able to discover how much food that takes. Your scale will be the most important piece of equipment in this experiment. You will read more about how to use Scream Weights in The 12 Tough Rules section.

Let Me Read Your Mind

Consider me psychic, but I know there is one last question burning in your brain. If thin people don't have great big metabolisms, what about that person you know (everyone knows one, it seems) who eats whatever he or she wants and remains permanently skinny?

I can't fully explain this phenomenon, other than to say that like other oddities such as mind reading and levitation there is usually a disappointingly mundane explanation for its occurrence. Often the skinny folks are still young (youth burns more) or smokers (smoking kills you in other ways, but prevents weight gain) or active men. Possibly this person eats less at other times or chooses foods that don't convert to fat as easily.

Having said this, though, we do know that responses to eating can differ and such a difference could explain your able-to-eat anything friend. This fact has been shown very clearly in a number of studies, including a well-known study of twins done by Dr. Claude Bouchard in 1990.

Dr. Bouchard took twelve pairs of male identical twins and overfed them by a total of 84,000 calories over 100 days. The subjects lived in a controlled environment so their intake could be observed. Here are the fascinating results. The average weight gain overall was eighteen pounds. Each twin gained pretty much the same weight as his brother did and put the extra pounds in just about the same area of his body. But the weight gain varied widely between twin pairs. One pair, for example, gained about nine and one-half pounds, while another gained twenty-nine pounds. Some twin pairs gained weight in the middle of the body, while others distributed

the pounds differently. In other words, there appeared to be a genetic difference in how different bodies used the same number of calories.

So, undoubtedly there are some people who can eat more than you
and not pay for it as dearly. Bummer.

If it makes you feel better, though, I can report that unregulated eating
catches up with pretty much everyone eventually. In 2007, the Framingham Heart Study issued a report on the probability of any individual in
their city becoming overweight or obese during a lifetime. Given current
rates of weight gain, the likelihood of Framingham's young and middle
aged citizens being overweight or obese in the long-term is predicted at
nine out of ten. In short, as time marches on, few "metabolic supermen"
will remain standing. If we do not monitor what we eat, the modern food
environment will defeat even the hardiest metabolism eventually.

Chapter Wrap

- Metabolism can be measured as the number of calories
  your body uses in a day.
- Your metabolism is created by the calories you burn at
  rest, the calories you use in moving around and the calories your body expends when digesting food.
- Most people have metabolisms that fall within predicted
  ranges for their size, age, and sex.
- Your metabolism is almost certainly within the normal
  range. The modern food world is not. Spend more time
  being angry at the destructive food world that surrounds
  you, and less time being angry at your body.
- Your metabolism is lower and slower now that you weigh
  less. This is normal. Be sure to eat appropriately less
  food in order to maintain weight. Do this by monitoring
  weight and eating to keep the scale stable.

Chapter Nine

Staying Afloat in the Food Flood

I have become increasingly convinced that many of the nutritional problems of Americans—not least of them obesity—can be traced to the food industry's imperative to encourage people to eat more in order to generate sales and increase income in a highly competitive marketplace.

—Marion Nestle, Ph.D., MPH, *Food Politics*

A cover article in *Business Week* magazine recently described strategies introduced by McDonald's to attract more customers. To make their restaurants more attractive, for example, the company had upscale café-style seating installed. They also erased some of the fast food atmosphere by installing ventilation systems which blew grease-laden smells out of the kitchen before they reached diners. The most profitable strategy for increasing business, though, turned out to be more basic—they decided to keep restaurants open around the clock. At the time the article was written, 40 percent of McDonald's franchises had gotten on the twenty-four-hour bandwagon and profits were soaring. McDonald's CEO, James Skinner, enthused, "We believe we've cracked the code in the United States. It's a simple secret, actually: Americans like to eat all day long. Having conquered lunch and dinner,...McDonald's plans to win the rest of the day."

Is McDonald's responsible for the obesity epidemic in our country? Certainly not—however, they and other major food sellers do shape our perceptions of "normal" eating—perceptions that are created through vast marketing activities. If restaurants are open round the clock, if food is available on every corner and in every television commercial, we soon feel that it is normal to eat continually.

The salesmen of Big Food are fond of claiming that they simply offer the product and it is your responsibility to choose wisely. But how can you choose well when you are constantly manipulated, stimulated, and assaulted by the presence of food?

Our modern eating environment is a food flood. Like a tsunami, the amount of food engulfing us every day is a disaster that leads to destruction and significant loss of life. You, the Maintenance Junior, are like a castaway on a small raft, tossed in that food-ridden sea. Most of those around you are going under, so you will need to look sharp!

How Do We Form Our Ideas About What to Eat?

Anthropologist Katherine Milton studies the history of food behaviors in primates. In comparing our eating styles to theirs, she writes, "Humans show little evidence of innate nutritional wisdom and individuals learn what to eat primarily through exposure to the eating habits of others. Until recently, most human societies ate time-tested diets, worked out over many generations by their ancestors. Today such traditional diets are largely a thing of the past...." In other words, humans aren't born knowing what to eat or when to stop. With traditional diets gone, our ideas about how to eat are entirely formed by the images and behaviors we see around us every day.

Immersion in any environment disables our ability to view it critically. In today's food world, we need to look past what passes for normal and ask: what is creating our ideas about how to eat?

For starters, it is easy to see that what passes for normal depends entirely on the time frame we examine.

Here is what was considered normal in the mid 1950s:

- Few restaurants
- Rare opportunities to eat out
- Minimal fast food (37 McDonald's nationally, 1 Burger King, no Wendy's)
- Most foods prepared from scratch at home
- Food sold mostly in small stores and markets
- Snacking between meals considered bad behavior
- Overweight kids uncommon (I still remember the names of the two kids I knew who were heavy)
- Size of a hamburger: 1 ounce
- Size of a drink: 8 ounces

Contrast that with what is considered normal in the early part of the 21st century:

- 54 billion meals sold at 844,000 restaurants each year in the U.S. alone
- 44 percent of American adults eating at a restaurant daily
- 31,000 McDonald's, 11,200 Burger King, 6,600 Wendy's worldwide
- Mc Donald's alone serving 46 million people each day
- Food omnipresent in locations like gas stations, pharmacies, and offices
- Childhood overweight common (The percentage of childhood overweight has quadrupled since 1970)
- Normal size of a hamburger: 6 oz
- Normal size of a drink: 24 oz

There is another important change in what we see as normal—the way we view ourselves. Research shows that we have come to see larger bodies as more acceptable than they used to be. Somewhere between one third and one half of men who are overweight or obese view their weight as normal.

When scientists recently asked overweight people how much weight they needed to lose, they were content to weigh significantly more than they would have been ten years earlier. We are rapidly moving toward seeing the overweight state as a normal condition of life.

In modern-day America, it is normal to eat out frequently, snack at will, order food to be delivered at home and consume desserts and treats. If these behaviors weren't normal, why would we have all those restaurants, food stores, food networks, food ads, and magazines devoted to cooking?

Because we have been led to believe that we can and should eat as we do, most overweight people come to the conclusion that there is something wrong with them personally—perhaps in their metabolism or genetics. But simple logic should tell us that if two thirds of us are overweight or obese, "normal" eating isn't working for anyone!

Who or what is responsible for the sea change in our view of food and of ourselves? Our environment is shaped by powerful forces,which urge us to eat. Most of these forces have little opposition. I believe it is important to your maintenance efforts that you identify them. These are the giants working against you.

Force One: Advertising

By far, the most frequent encouragements to eat come from those who sell food. The average child sees about 10,000 food ads per year on TV alone. If a parent resolved to lecture a child about healthy eating each day, this would only amount to 365 opposing messages. That's not much of a contest. At one time, the National Cancer Institute sponsored a program to push the health benefits of fruits and vegetables. They devoted $2 million to the effort. During the same period, Coke and Pepsi spent $3 billion on advertising their products. Which message got through? The total bill for food ads is around $30 billion per year and those ads are insidious and effective.

Force Two: Food availability

Food is everywhere. It is so everywhere that we don't even notice it anymore. Restaurant chains have convinced us that eating outside the home is simply a fact of life. And that message has worked. The amount of money Americans spend on fast food yearly has increased by $94 billion since the 1970s.

Food researcher Brian Wansink of Cornell makes a career of figuring out why people eat. In his book, *Mindless Eating*, Dr. Wansink's clever experiments show time and time again that the very nearness of easily available food provides an almost irresistible stimulus to eating.

Force Three: Seductive foods

Food manufacturers spend lots of time and energy on food engineering, the science of making foods more attractive to customers. A famous ice cream company, for example, has a well publicized flavor lab that constantly invents new, ever more seductive flavors. Coffeehouses have now come up with Banana Cream Frappucinos and other shake-like drinks that can contain hundreds of S Food calories. The constant reinvention of foods is strictly in the service of making them more saleable. Your health is generally not a consideration.

Force Four: The cost of "real" food

Fresh fruits and vegetables, fish, meat, and chicken are more expensive than fast food and/or packaged foods. This is one of the reasons that obesity is rampant in those with lower incomes. The ability to eat healthful foods has become a matter of economics.

Force Five: The food culture

As we discussed above, there is an overall acceptance of our modern way of eating. Few speak out against it, or even think about it much. Apart from the fact that food is everywhere, its prime role in our lives is expressed in other ways: chefs have become celebrities; entire TV channels are devoted to food and cooking; most newspapers have weekly food sections; huge numbers of cookbooks (and diet books) are produced yearly; cities sponsor chili cook-offs, rib burn-offs, and restaurant tastings, even when their populations are obese. I'm sure you can think of many other examples.

Force Six: Our increasingly overweight friends and family

Fascinating new data from the Framingham Heart Study reveals that a person who has a friend who becomes obese suffers a 57 percent greater chance of becoming obese himself. The spouse of an obese person has a 37 percent increased chance of becoming obese, and siblings of those who are obese have a 40 percent greater chance of meeting the same fate. Researchers feel that these results suggest a kind of person-to-person transmission of obesity. Perhaps, as obesity becomes more common in those you value, it may become more acceptable in yourself. You are also influenced by the behaviors of people around you. If they eat, you probably will too.

These factors shape the way we view "normal" eating and "normal" size. With overweight and obesity reaching critical levels, who is available to give a message of restraint and healthy eating? Here are the likely candidates:

Governmental Agencies—One would think that health agencies would provide valuable information about what to eat and act to oppose the unrestrained marketing of food. Unfortunately, the best-known source of federal diet guidelines is the USDA Food Pyramid. The U.S. Department of Agriculture, which produces the pyramid, is not a health agency. Its primary purpose is to represent American food production. In his excellent book, *Eat, Drink and Be Healthy*, Harvard professor Walter Willett describes how food lobbyists routinely pressure the USDA to alter food pyramid recommendations in order to get the best "spin" for their products. Our food pyramid is muddied by these conflicting interests and fails to give strong, independent guidance.

Honest efforts to promote accurate nutritional information are hampered by lack of funding. Food producers have vastly greater budgets for their products than the government has available for counter-messaging.

Despite the constant media attention to our obesity epidemic, government initiatives to address the problem are few and far between.

Our Schools—A good voice for health and nutrition? Unfortunately, schools often contribute to the problem rather than stand against it. The School Health Policies and Programs Study 2000, a national survey, observed that nearly every high school and the majority of middle schools in the U.S. contained food machines and/or soda machines. Over 40 percent of elementary schools let kids buy food and drinks on their own from machines and snack bars. Where it was once routine for school kids to attend daily gym class, only Illinois currently mandates daily physical activity in its schools. And despite that mandate, 74 percent of adults in Illinois are totally or partially sedentary.

The U.S. Department of Education reports that 99 percent of public schools have nutrition education, but that "the intensity and quality of the nutrition messages students are receiving is not known." Less than one third of schools provide information about motivation or eating behaviors. Further, education in nutrition drops off in high school, just at the time when eating disorders and confusion about eating begin to take hold.

The Media—Magazines that line the supermarket check-out aisle quote experts and offer endless articles about diet. Their covers are often frankly comical in their eagerness to display cakes and pies right alongside urgent pleas for weight loss. Magazine advice is, at best, suspect. I have an article on my desk which encourages dieters to choose white potato, popcorn, beer, cheese, and bagels as diet foods because they actually promote weight loss!

Magazines also tend to offer the same advice over and over again. I collect magazines which say "Walk Off the Weight!" on their cover. I add a new one to my stack nearly every week, yet no one seems to be getting any thinner.

It's become awfully hard to tell who the experts are. At one time, Mom was our nutrition expert, but now the job has passed to Dr. Phil, the Internet, and a thousand other sources. What was once obvious—what to eat—has become a big complicated mess.

The Medical Establishment—On the whole, doctors do a lackluster job of giving specific nutritional counseling. They are not trained to dispense this vital information and lack the necessary time.

Many doctors are also hesitant to discuss a patient's weight. In a study of over 12,000 overweight and obese people, 58 percent reported that their weight problem was never addressed by their primary care physician. This is especially unfortunate since other studies show that when a doctor suggests a patient lose weight, he or she is three times more likely to try.

Keeping Your Head Above Water

So how do you stay afloat in this food ocean? As you can see, there won't be much outside support, so you're going to need to craft your own rescue vehicle. You will stay afloat as long as you continue to see through the hype and keep your sights on the truth. To do this, I suggest you develop some righteous anger. When you're trying to do something difficult, it helps to get mad. As you learned earlier, athletes perform amazing feats by revving up their competitive juices. You can, too. Anger, properly applied, is motivating. It can keep you going through the tough times.

Here are some practical exercises for helping to see the food world as it really is. Each time you see it, get mad!

The U.S. Department of Agriculture, which produces the food pyramid, is not a health agency. Its primary purpose is to represent American food production.

• How much food did you eat on the days when you were losing your weight? The amount you ate then is not so very different from the amount of food you will need to stay thin. Visualize that day of food on a table. How much is it? Now, go into your local supermarket and look, really look, at the amount of food that is there. Is the purpose of your market to keep you healthy or is it to display, promote, and sell you food? Get mad!

• Pay close attention to the number of times you are "attacked" by food. By this I mean, how often is food brought to your attention when you don't wish it? Food Assault is occurring continually. Be aware of the pressures to eat that come from TV ads, radio jingles, check out line food displays, food in the office, food at the gas station, offers of food from friends, etc. Get mad!

• Watch food ads critically. Is that burger, that plate of fried shrimp, that ice cream sundae promoting the good health of the smiling person (always thin) who is eating it? Since the eating style these ads promote can lead to life-threatening illness, imagine that the foods being pushed are poisonous. View the ad through that lens and see how differently the message looks. Get mad!

• Look for the tricks that food makers use to get you to buy. Does the product have a homespun name? Is the packaging alluring? Is a celebrity touting the product? Is there a coupon or a giveaway? Are your kids being lured by a cartoon character? Does the product claim to have a miraculous health benefit? Remember that the foods you need to eat to stay at goal are "quiet"...no ads, no coupons, no claims. If a product is trying to get your attention, get mad!

• Pay close attention to the eating going on around you. Chances are you will be shocked at the food choices made by those you know. It's OK, and even helpful, to cultivate a little sense of nutritional superiority. With each day, you are getting healthier while most of those you know are taking a path toward illness. For their sake, get mad!

• Get especially mad for our kids!!! Who is teaching them about nutrition? Who is protecting them from the attack of food marketers? Who is there to prevent movies from linking themselves to fast food promotions and sugar-filled foods from representing themselves with cuddly cartoon characters? Who is encouraging them to move? Get mad!

• Pay close attention to the size of the people you see on the street. Obesity is driving up the cost of our medical care to an unprecedented degree, a cost that is passed along to every one of us who pays for health insurance. You may have resolved your personal problem, but you're still paying for the problem of others. People who eat without thinking are vastly driving up our collective health care bill. Get mad!

Chapter Wrap
• Our society's approach to eating appears to be normal, but is not. We know this because of the extensive disease burden that is linked to our modern diet.
• Most of what we hear and see will tend to convince us that eating as we do is perfectly fine.

Staying Afloat in the Food Flood

- To stay afloat in the flood of food, you will need to keep a close eye on your environment. Practice seeing the truth: our bodies need relatively small amounts of Primarian foods to stay healthy.
- There are powerful forces trying to push you into the ocean. Get mad to avoid being swept away with the tide!

Chapter Ten

Expect Sabotage

If you are not criticized, you may not be doing much.
  —Donald H. Rumsfeld, former U.S. Secretary of Defense

As you enter this new phase in your weight control saga, you will inevitably encounter sabotage. Unfortunately, saboteurs are often the people who are closest to Maintenance Juniors. They can be found among friends, family members, and coworkers.

In following a controlled food plan, you have stepped outside the general eating environment. You are no longer part of the club—and that will generate friction and negative comments. Despite the fact that these people care about you, they may do things to rattle your resolve.

Why does someone sabotage? There are probably many reasons, but the commonest would appear to be:

- **Anger.** Your new, controlled way of eating may be taken as an implicit criticism of the way friends and family eat.
- **Jealousy.** You look good and have control over a problem that others can't handle.
- **Fear.** Perhaps a significant change in your lifestyle will make you less accessible, no longer a part of the world in which your original relationship was formed. Perhaps, too, your new look may attract admiring glances from others.

Sabotage may be subtle or blatant. It may be hidden behind expressions of concern for health or it may be openly angry and challenging. In any of its forms, sabotage must be recognized and defused by Maintenance Juniors if they are going to succeed.

Recognizing the Many Forms of Sabotage

You will need to develop your sabotage detection mechanism. What should you be looking for?

Aggressive comments

One type of sabotage is the snide comment that relates to eating habits or size. Do any of the following sound familiar?

"Don't you know that the kind of diet you're eating isn't healthy?"

"You look much too thin."

"Don't you think it's a little crazy to watch everything you put in your mouth?"

"I hate being with people like you. You make me feel too guilty."

"You're taking this thing too far."

Each of these comments attempts to sway your behavior.

Spousal sabotage

Some of my married patients report being thrown off track by their spouses. Husbands may complain that Junior wives no longer bring the foods they like into the home or that they can't eat in places they used to enjoy.

Spouses may feel threatened by a partner's new size, particularly if they have their own weight issue. Encouraging regain is a way of establishing control over a partner whose new thinner self may be perceived as threatening to the relationship. Sabotage can take the form of insistence that S Foods and other altered foods be kept at home for the benefit of others in the family. It is difficult for Juniors to cook meals that totally depart from their own agendas, yet they are often asked to do just this by spouses.

One of my female patients is married to a man who has always been lean. He sabotages her efforts at weight control by insisting that junk food be kept at home and insists that since he can resist overeating it, she can as well. But she is a POW and he is a NOW. What with her physiology being quite different from his, she cannot.

Food assault

Saboteurs often use food assault as a weapon. This means offering and urging you to to eat food when you weren't even thinking about it. Since food is difficult to resist, this technique often works. Food assault by friends and family sounds like this:

Expect Sabatoge

"Come on! It's just one piece. That won't hurt you!!"

"You absolutely must try this. I made it just for you."

"It's a celebration. Have some!"

You will also experience a less personal type of food assault in your travels throughout our food culture. It's just assumed that you are part of the club—someone who eats indiscriminately. You will, therefore, be frequently asked to eat.

Just this morning I experienced food assault in my local coffeehouse. I asked for a skim milk latte. The young woman behind the counter then asked, "Would you like a muffin, a scone, or a sugar cookie with that?" When I politely refused, she tried again, "How about a piece of our carrot cake? It's really good." I said no. Her hand moved toward the register, then hung there. "A bagel?" she asked, hopefully. Three separate food assaults in under thirty seconds! I watched as she and her fellow salespeople worked this drill on each person in line. Not one customer had asked for anything more than coffee, but each was forced to say no to a load of S Food—a challenge that a number failed.

Workplace sabotage

Sabotage may be institutional. This happens when overeating is actually encouraged in the work environment.

One of our Maintenance Juniors works for a large corporation which claims to be very invested in employee health. She is constantly assaulted by corporate attempts to throw her off her eating plan. Candy bars are sent by management with notes that compliment employees on jobs well done. Corporate training sessions often use large jars of candy as rewards for learning, a technique more appropriate for Pavlov and his dog. The company sponsors "Pig Outs" and a weekly sweet day when each employee is assigned a turn at bringing in bakery treats.

This is an active kind of sabotage, one that directly invites people to eat. It makes little sense from a corporate perspective since such companies often struggle under the burden of health care costs incurred by their overweight employees.

A second kind of workplace sabotage is more subtle. It consists of the quiet, but constant, presence of food in the office, what I call "Second Hand Food." Just as secondhand smoke weakens the resolve of a recovered smoker, secondhand food forces maintainers into unwanted contact with a substance they are trying to avoid. At one time, office food was confined to a kitchen or break room. Now, many companies look the other way when employees eat while working. Desktops may offer candies, cakes and other snacks.

I have several patients who work in physicians' offices where pharmaceutical reps routinely provide lavish staff lunches. It is impossible for these maintainers to avoid exposure to this secondhand food, its smells and temptations. Worse, these Juniors say that their coworkers are generally unsympathetic. Those who are not struggling with weight often say they have a right to eat as they like. But should that right trump someone else's right to stay healthy? Whose claim is more valid? Since there is no good answer, the Maintenance Junior's best bet is to strongly defend his or her right to stay slim. Some strategies to do so are offered below.

Sabotage by failed dieters and maintainers

Sabotage often comes from those who have failed to lose or maintain weight loss themselves. Since this describes 80 to 95 percent of dieters, this creates quite a pool of potential saboteurs!

Melissa P., a Junior in our program, works with a woman who had bariatric surgery but regained most of her weight. This woman brings home-baked cookies and cakes to work constantly and insists on offering them around. She is especially persistent with those who are trying to lose weight. Baked goods are displayed throughout the day on her desk.

On one particular day, this woman asked Melissa to name her favorite dessert. Melissa said "Red Velvet Cake," but made it clear that she didn't eat it any longer due to her struggles with weight. The very next day, the saboteur appeared with a freshly baked version of Melissa's Achilles heel. When Melissa firmly stated that she preferred not to see or be exposed to the cake, her coworker walked past her desk and "flashed" the cake by lifting the foil wrapping.

Healthcare sabotage?

The strangest and saddest case of sabotage I know is the story of a patient who came to us with diabetes, high blood pressure, and elevated cholesterol. He lost 60 pounds and reversed each one of his medical problems. After the weight loss, he scheduled a visit with his cardiologist. He was very excited about going and showing off his incredible achievement. The great day came. The cardiologist entered the room, glanced at the patient and sniffed, "You lost the weight?

So, what? You'll just gain it all back." My patient was devastated. Certain that weight regain was inevitable, he returned to old habits and quickly fulfilled his doctor's prophecy.

Defusing Sabotage

Sabotage will most certainly happen, so learn to handle it. It is a good idea to have stock responses for those who make comments about the way you eat.

Responding to comments about your eating style

Saboteur: "Why don't you eat the bread? That's crazy."

Your Response: "I'm on a special medical program that prohibits starches and sugars for now. Wish I could join you, but by all means you go ahead and enjoy."

(This allows others at the table to eat bread, starch, and dessert without guilt. They will probably pity you a bit. But that's OK.)

Saboteur: "You look awful. That weight loss makes you look older."

Your Response: "I didn't do this for my looks. I did it for my blood pressure and cholesterol. Thank goodness they're normal now."

Saboteur: "It's crazy to watch everything that you eat the way you do. Can't you just eat moderately?"

Your Response: "I wish I could, but that just hasn't worked for me in the past and this does."

Saboteur: "The idea that you'll never eat bread or pasta is crazy."

Your Response: "Vegetarians never eat meat and no one seems to think that's strange."

Responding to cake flashing
and other aggressive workplace sabotage

As a first step, speak directly to the offenders and ask that food be kept out of sight. If that fails, ask your office supervisor to restrict food to areas that you can avoid. Ask for help politely, but be sure to emphasize the great importance of your weight loss to your health. If you have improved or cured such conditions as blood pressure, cholesterol, or diabetes—say so. These changes are saving your employer significant dollars in health care costs. Be creative, insistent, and proactive. Write letters to managers and directors that make them aware of the negative impact of workplace eating on employee health.

You are one of the first soldiers in the battle for a food-free work environment. As more and more of us lose weight, it will become increasingly common to ask that others remove food from the office. Eventually, and with your help, food-free workspaces will become as politically correct as smoke-free workspaces.

Responding to spousal sabotage

This may help:

> "I am following this maintenance plan so that I can be around to support and love you for years to come. I'm doing it for you! So please help me out. To do this, I can't be around foods that trigger my appetite. Let's work out a way that I don't have to see these foods. You can eat whatever you want outside of our home, but within it, we're going to have to stay Primarian."

Chapter Wrap

- Sabotage is to be expected. In fact, sabotage tells you that you've done a good job with weight loss and maintenance and that others notice.
- Be sure to identify it for what it is, take pride in your accomplishments and defuse it as soon as possible.

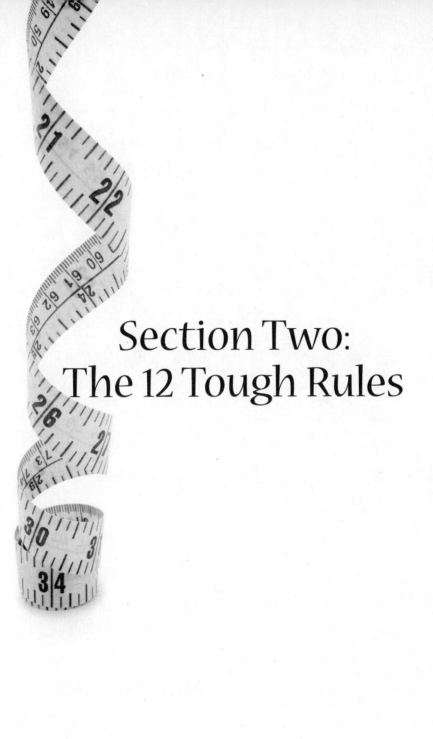

Section Two:
The 12 Tough Rules

Chapter Eleven

The 12 Tough Rules

Rule 1: Be Tough, Not Moderate

Rule 2: Commit Yourself to a Three Month Opt Out Period

Rule 3: Weigh Yourself Every Day

Rule 4: Reverse Small Regains Immediately

Rule 5: Eat Primarian 90 Percent of the Time

Rule 6: Eat One Major Meal Per Day

Rule 7: Perform a Daily "Scan and Plan"

Rule 8: Stop Eating at 8 P.M.

Rule 9: Eat from a Limited Menu

Rule 10: Have One Acceptable Treat per Day

Rule 11: Have a Love Affair with Exercise

Rule 12: Maintain with Support and Support Others

Rule 1: Be Tough, Not Moderate

Conventional wisdom about maintaining weight counsels us to return to life as before, only to do things in moderation. Unfortunately, experience shows that this type of moderate approach doesn't work. For this reason, Rule 1 asks you to forget compromises and take a tough stance.

Why is gastric bypass surgery such an effective fix for obesity? The reason is simple. It is not moderate. Surgery creates, and permanently enforces, a drastic change in food intake. The reduced stomach size makes you sick if you eat too much and the intestinal rerouting causes malabsorption further down the line. This is drastic indeed. And effective.

People Magazine periodically runs a popular feature called "Half Their Size." Each issue highlights the stories of people who have lost large amounts of weight and are maintaining successfully. What is interesting is that their approaches are far from moderate. Here are some of the exercise habits reported by maintainers in past issues:

- Swims an hour a day
- Walks up to ten miles a day
- Works out on treadmill and uses weights for an hour six days a week
- Teaches karate to kids and is working toward a black belt
- Works as a personal trainer

And here are a few of the meals these maintainers report eating:

- slice diet bread, 1 boiled egg, 1 apple
- 20 almonds, ½ pound broccoli
- 2 cups steamed vegetables, 8 medium shrimp, and 2 sesame crackers

These are not little tweaks to previous behaviors. Senior Level Maintainers like these know that small changes in behavior don't lead to the big results they want.

Here's the lesson: deep, major changes work when it comes to keeping weight off. To embrace significant change as the only road to permanent success, follow the steps below.

Rule 1, Step One:
Avoid moderation strategies

A "moderation strategy" is an eating plan that asks you to make small, painless changes but promises big, exciting results. This kind of wishful thinking is very seductive but—like getting something for nothing—it turns out to be too good to be true.

If the cultural forces that overwhelm us with food are like a flood, we must respond in kind. Putting our faith in moderate approaches is akin to relying on an umbrella to ward off a tsunami. We live in an extremely *immoderate* food environment. As a result, the use of half-hearted defenses dooms us to certain failure.

Having said this, how can we recognize a moderation strategy? Here are some of these strategies and the reason each is ineffective:

• **Eliminate one food item from your diet each day. At the end of a year, all those little calories will add up to big weight loss.**

How often have you read this one? And how many people do you know who have lost weight this way? On its face, this plan seems reasonable. Eating two fewer chocolate chip cookies each day should cause a daily deficit of 120 calories. That adds up to 43,800 calories saved per year, or twelve and one-half pounds lost! Looks good on paper, but it doesn't work in practice.

Perhaps if each of us ate exactly the same number of calories every day and burned exactly the same amount, such a cutback might work. But we don't do either. The two cookies we eliminate get made up by a few bites of another food somewhere else in your day. Your body is easily able to compensate for small changes made to your diet.

• **Eat only when you are truly hungry.**

Maintenance Juniors often tell me they plan to try this moderation strategy. Unfortunately it, too, fails to work. Why? Because true hunger is impossible to distinguish from false hunger. Our hungry feelings are complicated biological phenomena that are often triggered just by being near food. In a world where food is so plentiful, few of us are ever in desperate need of calories—true hunger. Yet we often feel very real feelings of hungriness and want to eat. These stomach rumblings can be brought on by the time of day, the location in which we find ourselves (like our kitchens and offices), and most commonly from direct exposure to food itself. At such times we don't physically need food, yet the hormones that are released and the feelings they create are certainly real. How can we sort out which of our many hunger feelings are the legitimate ones? We can't.

• **Eat until you're full and no more.**

This would seem to be an easy solution except for the fact that fullness turns out to be annoyingly relative. A recent research study by Brian Wansink at Cornell University proved this point. Pairs of participants were asked to eat a bowl of soup. One participant had a normal soup bowl, while the second was given a rigged bowl that refilled itself as the soup was consumed. Dr. Wansink found that those whose bowls refilled themselves ate 73 percent more soup but felt no fuller than their partner eaters. They didn't even know that they had eaten more. This research confirms the fact that our eyes and our stomachs are wired together. When we see food, we are hungry and we may not feel full until it disappears from view.

• Eat anything you want, just do it in moderation.

This is the quintessential moderation strategy. It is the mantra of most maintainers and the most repeated maintenance belief. Unfortunately, I believe it leads to failure. Why doesn't this simple strategy work?

It assumes that any of us can figure out what moderate is. We have been used to eating so excessively in our lifetimes, that what most of us consider to be moderate consumption is far too much food to maintain lost weight.

It also makes no distinction between food types, which often have very different addictive or hunger producing potentials. S Foods, as you already know, make people hungry and are extremely easy to overconsume. While it may be possible to eat salmon and apples moderately, it simply may not be possible to do the same with bread, pasta, chips, or cookies.

Remember the Lay's potato chip slogan, "Bet you can't eat just one"? There's a reason that tag-line had a ring of truth. Most people find themselves quickly re-addicted to S Foods and consuming more and more each day.

Rule 1, Step Two:
Make peace with the word "diet."

Recently, *The New York Times* bemoaned the fate of a woman who had undergone gastric bypass surgery some years before:

> "...170 pounds lighter than when she started, she still needs to restrict her food intake to keep from gaining it all back. Even with the surgery, and even maintaining a weight that is bor-derline obese...*she can never enjoy food with complete and carefree abandon.*" (italics mine.)

We are in trouble if we think that weight loss or bariatric surgery will magically allow us to eat with "complete and carefree abandon." POWs will always be sensitive to the modern eating environment so it helps to make peace with the word "diet," not deny its existence. To make a start, let's restructure the way we look at this much maligned word.

A diet is simply a program for eating. It needn't have anything to do with weight. It does, however, have everything to do with planning and control. There are vegetarian diets, low salt diets, macrobiotic diets, Mediterranean diets, gluten-free diets, and scores of others, all based on personal beliefs about eating and health.

Choosing to follow a diet is a good thing. It means that you have a thoughtful philosophy about the

Here's the lesson: deep, major changes work when it comes to keeping weight off.

food world. It means that you are looking critically at the foods around you and are making decisions based on your beliefs. As we have said repeatedly, difficult tasks are never accomplished without clear planning. More than anything else, Maintenance Juniors need regimentation and a strategy. A diet provides both. So, now is not the time to throw away diet. Now is the time to construct your lifelong diet.

Rule 1, Step Three:
Establish a life charter

Let's call this permanent eating plan your life charter. A life charter must be based on your beliefs about food and health. Your greatest job as a Junior is to create this plan and refine it so that it fits your tastes. This plan is like a government's constitution. It is based on principles and rules, but should be basic enough that its framework can be easily committed to memory. Portability and ease of use are key. Once you establish your life charter, you should be able to consult it mentally to locate the guidelines for any eating situation.

As an example, let me share my own charter with you. Mine is based on my belief in eating scarcely and in consuming a Primarian diet. It is constructed to keep me at a low, healthy weight based on my belief that lower weights convey the best lifelong health outcomes. My charter also reflects my belief that healthy nutrition can only work in the setting of a body that runs well, and therefore includes a commitment to exercise.

The primary goal of my charter is to achieve the longest possible life in the best possible health, hopefully avoiding periods of illness or disability as I age. A secondary goal, important to me personally, is to properly honor the gift of life I have been given and to appreciate the miraculous nature of my body by treating it with utmost respect.

Here is my life charter:

1. I eat one major meal per day, and 90 percent of my diet is Primarian.
2. I eat starches and sugars extremely rarely.

3. I eat one allowable treat daily (more if the scale cooperates).
4. I eat processed foods extremely rarely.
5. I eat no trans fats and very few saturated fats.
6. I honor my body by not allowing junk foods to enter it.
7. When I gain weight, I immediately reduce to below Scream Weight.
8. I work out vigorously six days per week.

My plan is utterly portable and has become second nature. When I am invited to a wedding, I know that I will be skipping any fatty cuts of meat (saturated fat) and the wedding cake (modern starch and sugar plus saturated fat). I will have eaten lightly for the rest of the day because I will have planned the wedding dinner as my one major meal. If I'm hungry after the party, I know I can have my one allowable treat, usually a good sized dish of low-fat ice cream.

What about bread, grains, pasta, corn, rice, and potatoes? I am 90 percent Primarian, which gives me the option to indulge in these very occasionally. The longer I spend as a Primarian, though, the less I want to deviate. I am usually aware that I can have a piece of bread if I really want it, but I almost always opt out. I think that you will be surprised at how much easier food choice becomes when you have absolute guidelines.

Resolve not to be swayed by what others are eating or by their comments. Just as a vegetarian does not eat roast beef simply because others at the table are chowing down, so you must learn to rely on the wisdom of your life charter. Be proud of your plan and make every attempt to follow it staunchly. Many vegetarians avoid meat to protect the rights of animals and to spare them unnecessary suffering. Their motives in following an alternative diet are not questioned, nor should yours be. Remember that you have an equally noble goal: to preserve a human body's optimal health and function (yours!)

Despite all the ideas about eating I've suggested, your charter may turn out looking very different from mine. I don't ask you to accept every idea I put forth, but rather to see what works for you and to follow your charter faithfully, daily, and not moderately.

Rule 1, Step Four:
Accept the drug-like nature of S Foods and avoid them

It would be lovely if we could return to eating crackers, bread, cake, and candy while simply controlling our intake. Perhaps, one day, a really terrific drug will make all that possible. That day is not yet here. The idea of eating just a little bit of modern food ignores an enormous problem. Modern S Foods are addictive.

In Chapter Seven, we discussed the parallel between drugs and S Foods. Consider the similarities:

- **S Foods induce cravings.** Most of us have cravings for modern S Foods (rarely for fish, vegetables or fruit, you might notice).
- **S Foods create pleasure.** Eating sweets and starches gives us a pleasurable "food high."
- **Stopping S Foods causes a sense of withdrawal.** When we begin a diet, there is an unpleasant period of hunger and withdrawal that lasts days or more after modern foods are eliminated.
- **S Foods are difficult to control.**

When we reintroduce exposure to these foods, a small amount often causes us to fall off the wagon.

Remember that familiar advice to eat whatever you like...just in moderation? If you are willing to agree that there are many similarities between addictive drugs and modern foods, you must next ask yourself: would anyone ever give a drug addict the advice to just use drugs moderately?

You may well object to this analogy. After all, you might say, drugs are highly potent substances that are nearly impossible to control and S Foods are not nearly as dangerous or as addictive. I would argue differently. S Foods are very harmful when ingested by people who don't process them well (POWs). S Foods become dangerous when the fat they cause leads to serious medical problems. In addition, S Foods may actually be tougher to control than drugs. Here's why:

- The use of S Foods is idealized, glamorized and encouraged by major corporations. S Food products are advertised on every TV channel, magazine page, and billboard. Their use is linked with pleasure and well-being. Drugs are not advertised, encouraged or condoned in any public forum.
- There are stores that sell S Foods on every corner and opportunities to buy S Foods at vending machines and in

non-food locations like gas stations. Purchasing drugs is still difficult and furtive.

- On Valentine's Day, your lover sends you a box of sugary treats to show his or her devotion—not drugs.
- We celebrate happy occasions with plates piled high with S Foods—not drugs.
- No one brings boxes of drugs to work each day to tempt users in break-rooms and on desks. But they do bring doughnuts, bagels, chips, and candy.

Which substance is the tougher one to avoid? Which one is tied in our mind to love, happiness, and well-being? While the addictive powers of drugs may be stronger than those of food, the incredible flood of food in which we operate makes S Food addiction nearly unavoidable and extremely difficult to kick.

Rule 1, Step Five:
Practice, practice, practice

How do you get to Carnegie Hall? To master any skill, try and try again. To do this, make a personal game of negotiating tough food situations. Go into them with a plan ("I'll hold the vegetable hors d'oeuvres in one hand, and nurse a single glass of wine in the other") and a goal ("I'm going to figure out how I can enjoy this wedding without eating the cake.") One successful maintainer told me that she diverts herself from food at parties by vowing to learn five things about each guest she meets. This has not only kept her weight off, but has provided the opportunity to have some fascinating conversations she would have otherwise missed.

You can't become an expert maintainer until you have faced challenges and learned how to prevail. So don't be afraid to go to dinners, out to parties, to conferences, and to events. Rely on your cleverness and strength. The more successes you have, the more you will be convinced of your ability to succeed long-term.

Rule 1 in a nutshell

- Adopt a tough maintenance strategy using the 12 Tough Rules.
- Don't fear the challenge; take a warrior's attitude.
- Practice your strategy by putting yourself in situations that would normally tempt you to eat.

- Establish (and doggedly follow) your life charter.
- Never let others dictate your eating plan.
- Have pride in the battle you are waging.
- Absolutely refuse to deviate or be deviated from your plan.

Rule 2: Commit Yourself to a Three-Month Opt Out Period

Now that you have learned Rule 1, it's time to bring your toughness to bear on your first real challenge. As you start your new maintenance plan, I will ask you to strive for three perfect months. Perfect technique in maintenance is defined as:

- Following each of the 12 Tough Rules without deviation.
- Eating only Primarian foods, with the exception of your one allowable treat.
- Working on an active remodeling of your life.

I call this three-month "detox" the opt out period.

Like the "Force" in Star Wars, our eating habits have both a light side and a dark side. The light side means enjoyable eating of pleasurable, nourishing foods. The dark side means binging, eating addictively, and choosing foods that destroy health. For three months, my aim is to bring you out of the dark, allowing you to gain balance, steadiness, and wisdom. This training will give you an edge against the Darth Vader side of food. At the same time, three months in a world without modern eating will teach you to enjoy a food freedom that you have not yet known. Remember that it's just a three-month commitment out of a long life!

You need time to break up with your old diet

Your old eating habits are like a dysfunctional relationship with a partner you love, but just can't live with. What happens when you break up? First, you mourn. You think about all the good times you had. You resist the urge to call. You almost pick up the phone.

If you stay tough, the memories fade and the hurting stops. Time heals and life goes on. Eventually, you find someone else—someone who treats you better.

On the other hand, if you make that call and keep going back just "one more time," you're back in the thick of it before you know it.

The three-month opt out period is your opportunity to break-up with the Western diet. During this time, don't play with the modern foods that got you into trouble. Mourn a little and let them go! Pretty soon, life will take on another shape and your new eating partner will start to feel pleasurable. Want to learn to actually prefer that change? You can, as long as you resist the temptation to place a late night call to your old flame.

You are vulnerable right now, so be careful

Right now, you are especially vulnerable to your trigger foods and they can easily get the upper hand. Here's why:

- Lots of people are encouraging you to eat trigger foods now that you're thinner.
- You were hoping to get a reward for successful dieting (that usually means food).
- You crave a return to the "real world."

My plan, as radical as it may sound, asks you to toughen up just when you'd most like to give in. I have faith in you. The first three months of maintenance is a time to clean house and utterly remake your food priorities. If, after this period, you are as happy with your renovated life as I think you will be, you may want to adopt a completely Primarian style of eating permanently. If not, you can look forward to adding back small amounts of the foods you've missed as you move past the opt out period.

Life without S Foods seems bleak at first glance...it really isn't. Life without S Foods seems depriving...but turns out not to be. Eating Primarian would appear to be a recipe for constant hunger. Just the opposite is true. If you give yourself a chance to adapt to a new, genetically consistent diet, you will find that you no longer crave trigger foods and that your hunger level is much more controlled. I can attest to this personally because I have been a Primarian for five years. Once you have reached this happy stage, your battle with food and weight can truly be won. But you must give yourself a chance, and that means commiting to a real attempt to follow the rules.

Why a three-month opt out?

Three months is the minimum time period for detoxing your diet. I know most people cannot accept the idea of a life without ever having a slice of pie or a piece of bread. While I would dearly love to see all of you change your menus completely, the three month opt out will empower you to exert a control over occasional deviations that you now lack.

Once the first three months are past, you can add a few S Foods back to your diet if you really want to. But I caution you to remain very wary of them, and only do so if you are feeling in control. You can read more about adding back under Tough Rule 5. For now, let's move on to the steps that will guarantee a successful opt out period.

Rule 2, Step One:
Drop "cheat" and substitute "choice"

When patients tell me that they fell off their diets, they like to confess with a sly smile that they "cheated." To me, it sounds as if they're saying something quite different: "Take that, Diet Doc! I broke your rules."

Even though it was your idea to get thin and stay that way, it's easy to start thinking of the changes you need to make as a burden that's being imposed on you. You get a little revenge (against the world, your genes, maybe this book?) by cheating. I don't have to tell you that this is ultimately self-defeating.

Long term changes in diet must come from you and only you. Whether you follow the rules laid out in this book or an utterly different strategy, you must sign on to the program and make it yours. Then, if you deviate, it's not cheating—it's having a plan that's not working.

Failures need attention and your strategy needs a rethinking. I would much prefer that you said, "I just couldn't make things work this week" or "I made a choice and I've got to deal with it" than "I cheated." Getting rid of that phrase when you lapse will help you take responsibility for the plan you've chosen.

Rule 2, Step Two:
Add while subtracting

During the opt out period and throughout your Junior year, you are going to feel deprived at times. You can help overcome this by adding things to compensate for that feeling of subtraction. Do this by working on building a new persona for yourself.

Each of our lives is like a table supported by a sturdy set of legs. For most of us, the legs that hold us steady include our primary relationships, our careers, and the things that give us pleasure. Modern foods can form a large part of that last leg. Dietary change that excludes "thrill eating" yanks out that support. If the other legs holding us up are not firm, or if pleasurable things other than eating don't exist for us, our table may collapse.

Even assuming the rest of your life is in good balance, taking away a major pleasure leaves your stool a bit shaky. That is why, during the opt out period, I ask you to create new pleasures and supports—in other words—to add while you subtract. The most valuable addition is a greater focus on athleticism, but more on that later. There are many other things you can do as well. These are just a few suggestions:

Change your exterior:
Adopt a new style of clothing.
Switch to a completely different hairstyle.
Do away with your old makeup routine and find a new one.
Whiten your teeth.
Get new glasses or contact lenses.
Change your hair color.

Change your interior:
Learn a new language.
Write the story or book you've always wanted to get on paper.
Start playing an instrument.
Read a series of books.
Take a class in something you've longed to learn.
Join a performing arts group.

Change your environment:
Remove all the clutter from your house.
Rearrange your furniture.
Plant a garden.
Remodel, repaint, repaper.
Downsize.

Change your spirit:
Meditate.
Learn yoga, tai chi, or another spiritual practice.
Take solitary walks in silence.
Reconnect with your religious traditions.

Devote time to a cause that helps those in need.

Become politically active.

Work on truly revising and recreating yourself. In this way, you will not just be restricting what you eat. Your eating style will just be part of the larger change you are making.

Rule 2, Step Three:
Think strategically

The opt out period calls for strategy. Here are some behaviors that work for people, but don't be afraid to come up with your own.

- **Search for primary foods that really do it for you.**

There are dozens of varieties of apples, pears, and oranges alone.

Experiment with fruit and vegetable types that are new to you. Try odd combinations like fruit on top of traditional salads. Put mustard on an apple! Eat pears and salsa! Get creative.

- **Cultivate a lifelong habit of attentional eating.**

Every time you begin to eat something, draw back for a moment and decide if that food honors you body. If it is primary and unadulterated and fits into your daily plan, it is something that adds to you and your health.

- **Observe others closely.**

You will be amazed at what people around you are eating. Feel free to (silently) indulge in feelings of diet superiority.

- **Wear revenge clothes.**

I don't know exactly why I call your "thin" clothes Revenge Clothes, but my patients seem to understand what I mean. Maybe it's because the nice, snug clothes that fit you now are your way of saying "Ha!! I did it!" to the world. Wear the clothes that show off your new size proudly, and don't revert to the temptation to hide in your baggy jeans. Wearing revenge clothes to events where food temptations are likely will help you to avoid choosing the wrong things.

- **Keep meals simple and reduce exposure time to foods.**

Things will be dicey for the first three months, so your best bet is to keep face-time with food to a minimum. Keep your house clear of S

Foods. If this is not possible, ask family members to keep them in a spot where you won't easily encounter them. Prepare meals that are easy and quick until you are firmly anchored in maintenance.

Not perfect?

What if this three-month plan doesn't work for you? Remember two things: First, no single eating plan works for every person. Don't give up. Try modifying things to fit your needs. You don't have to listen to everything I say just because it's in a book. Adapt the things that work for you and discard the things that don't. Or try another strategy entirely. Second, most successful long-term maintainers have failed several times before achieving permanent success. In other words, it takes a while to get maintenance right. Whether this is your first try at anchoring your weight or your hundred and first, a detailed plan will make the difference.

For successful maintainers, the end of the three month opt out period will have brought a change in how they see food. This is not to say that struggles won't continue. But they will be less intense. One of my most consistent maintainers likes to refer to herself as a "weight loss survivor." She says that she will always see her life through the lens of what she was: a heavy person with an addictive relationship to food. The difference now is that she has ended her relationship with the foods that made her fat. Her struggles with eating are controllable and she is proud of her daily successes.

Rule 2 in a nutshell
- Try your level best to opt out of the modern eating world and maintain a completely Primarian diet for three months.
- Find ways to enjoy your new eating plan.
- Work on a self-remodeling, including interior and exterior renovations, so that you can add while subtracting.
- Don't beat yourself up when you slip. Just rededicate yourself to your efforts.

Making the Scale Work for You

Rule 3: Weigh Yourself Every Day

If you have ever tried to count calories, figure out the precise percent of fat or carbs in your day, or stay in some exactly calculated food zone, you know that these strategies for eating are impossible to sustain for very long. For weight maintenance, the two best and most effective principles are: eat from a Primarian menu and respect the scale.

Your scale is the most important piece of equipment in your life as a weight maintainer. Weighing every day will allow you to make the small changes in your diet that you need to stay at goal. Weighing every day will quickly show you the unique responses of your body to various foods. Since each of us is different, this is information that each must learn through personal experience. Your scale can help you do this.

Recent scientific data strongly supports the effectiveness of daily weighing during maintenance. In October 2006, a lead study in the *New England Journal of Medicine* described a trial involving 314 people who had lost an average of about forty pounds each. Study participants who were taught to weigh daily and to make corrections based on this weight, maintained significantly more effectively. Those who were assigned to a combination of daily weighing and supportive counseling did best. This is the reason I will ask you to continue to seek help throughout maintenance with Tough Rule 12.

Recruiting the scale as your best friend makes things simple. This is how it works: eat as much as you can from a Primarian menu while trying to stay within goal range. Immediately institute a prearranged plan for weight reversal when you exceed goal.

Rule 3, Step One:
Weigh properly

Weigh yourself only once per day—in the morning, without clothes. Do not weigh later in the day as weight fluctuates greatly in later hours as the result of fluid shifts and changes in elimination. Weighing late in the day is a recipe for frustration and disaster, so make sure that your weight is checked only in the morning. If you miss a morning weigh-in, skip that day.

Be unflinching. If you fell off plan and ate seven tacos and a milkshake the night before, weigh anyway. Remember, you are a scientist collecting data and the most valuable information is that which you discover after messing up. Many POWs are afraid of looking at the scale. If that's you, get over the fear and see that little platform as an irreplaceable tool for learning about yourself. Before long, it will be difficult to get out of bed without heading for that familiar spot.

Rule 3, Step Two:
Use the right equipment

The kind of scale you choose is unimportant as long as it is consistent. I recommend a digital scale that weighs in tenths of a pound. This will help you see small deviations. Little fluctuations are not that vital, but give you a sense of how your weight changes from day to day. Fancy scales that include body fat and water measurements have more information than you need. Don't get hung up on other numbers. Sticking to monitoring weight is enough. Remember, too, that scales outside your home may weigh quite differently from yours. If you weigh yourself somewhere else, take this into account. Don't get overly concerned if the weight is higher than what you get on your home scale. It is the consistency of weight from day to day and not the absolute number that we're looking for.

Rule 3, Step Three:
Weigh bravely and daily

Your success in maintenance revolves around balancing the relationship between you and your scale. This provides an easy method for maintaining. You will not need counting or calculating of nutrient grams or percents. In fact, I discourage this. If you eat following the principles outlined in Chapters Five and Six, your nutritional needs will be well cared for.

With general nutrition out of the way, the next order of business is to figure out how much volume you can eat. To do this, simply weigh yourself daily and watch for fluctuations. There will be many.

Body weight is dependent on numerous factors including salt intake, sweat and elimination, hormonal shifts and—seemingly—the phases of the moon. If you are losing weight, eat more Primarian foods. If you are staying pretty much in one weight range with a few fluctuations up and down, continue eating as you are doing. Eat as much as you can from your Primarian menu while keeping your weight stable. Attempt to find a way to feel nicely nourished, and not deprived.

Rule 3, Step Four:
Don't count calories

I know that it seems like heresy to make this suggestion, but let me clarify my reasoning. As part of my intake interview with new patients, I ask each how he or she has successfully lost weight in the past. Virtually no one has ever referenced calorie counting as a way they have taken off pounds. The reason? Counting is burdensome.

It is also inaccurate. A number of studies have shown that neither dieters nor diet "experts" can count calories accurately. In one New York University study, for example, 203 dietitians were asked to estimate the calorie and fat content of five restaurant meals—including lasagna, a grilled-chicken Caesar salad, and a tuna-salad sandwich. Despite their expertise, they underestimated the calories by an average of 37 percent and the fat by 49 percent. Among other errors, they guessed the tuna sandwich had about 375 calories when it actually contained 720 calories. Why should you assume that you will be able to do any better than a trained dietician?

Watching the scale is a way of forcing calories to stay in a reasonable range without tallying them. Focusing on the type of food you choose, rather than its calorie content will be more valuable to you in the end.

Rule 3 in a nutshell

- As a Maintenance Junior, you are a scientist collecting fascinating data about yourself.
- Your major source of data comes from your scale.
- Use fluctuations to adjust intake.
- Weigh daily and learn.

How to Use a Scream Weight

Rule 4: Reverse Small Regains Immediately

Of the many terms I've made up for my patients, "Scream Weight" is my favorite. For Juniors, Scream Weight is the scale number you never want to see—ever again. If that number appears, flashing in digital red, you shriek! Reaching Scream Weight should trigger an immediate response—man the battle stations and take action.

Rule 4, Step One:
Set your scream weight

Pick a personal Scream Weight and monitor yourself to stay below it. This weight should sit five to eight pounds higher than the new weight you achieved with weight loss. If possible, your Scream Weight should be at a tens transition. For example, if you have reduced to 144, set your Scream Weight at 150. In practice, this appears to confer a slight mental advantage. Increasing your weight from 149 to 150 may represent a gain of just one pound, but it moves you from the 140s to the 150s, packing a greater psychological punch. It is possible to set Scream Weights at fives (for example a weight of 160 and a Scream Weight of 165), but be advised that they may not work quite as well.

Rule 4, Step Two:
Adjust scream weight if necessary

You may not be able to determine the weight you truly want to maintain until you have been on a Primarian diet for a month or more. Some post-dieters (particularly those who have been on a very restrictive plan or have achieved quite low weights) will gain five to ten pounds after they begin eating freely. If this has happened to you, it is fine to accept this new weight and set your Scream Weight at a higher level than the one you originally chose. A modest initial regain seems to represent a replenishing of body stores. Don't panic. You may find it easier to maintain permanently once this upward adjustment has occurred. Be realistic and set a maintenance weight that you can live with rather than a dream weight that makes you miserable. The same may be said for later stages of maintenance. If it is an impossible battle to anchor at the weight you'd hoped for, move your Scream Weight up a bit.

Rule 4, Step Three:
Observe weight swings carefully

Many Juniors will be surprised to find that, at least at the beginning, they reach Scream Weight as often as once a week. This is normal. As I've already said, there are many reasons for weight to go up and down. One of the reasons we haven't yet discussed is the body's tendency to use and refill stores of glycogen. Glycogen is a sugary back-up pack of ready energy that is kept in the muscles and liver. Just as the battery in your laptop takes over when the computer is not plugged in, glycogen acts as a portable energy source when you are not eating food.

Glycogen is composed of chains of sugar, which are stored in combination with water. This water makes glycogen heavy. As your body burns the stored sugar for fuel, water is freed up and eliminated.

In the first week of your weight loss diet, you may remember that you spent a lot of time in the bathroom. Because you had vastly cut down on eating, your body was burning up most of its glycogen and jettisoning all the attached water.

Glycogen is a vital part of our energy balance system, but its heaviness can be an annoyance for maintainers. Normal fluxes in the amount you have on board may change your weight by a number of pounds in either direction. Each unit of glycogen weighs more than an equivalent unit of fat. Since glycogen stores are continually in flux, it is normal for weight to trend up and down.

Slipping up with S Foods (which become sugars, as you remember) will give your body large supplies of glucose to store as glycogen. With the addition of the requisite water, this glycogen will make you pay on the scale. This is one reason Juniors often find they have gained two or more pounds the morning after a binge with pasta, bread or dessert. Another reason is that carbohydrate, and the insulin it stimulates, causes the kidneys to hold onto salt and water. This means that you retain fluid.

Rule 4, Step Four:
Put it in reverse

The key to using Scream Weight is to train yourself to immediately reverse small regains. You will need to correct your course with frequent changes of direction. To do this, set up a plan for cutting back on days when your scale approaches Scream Weight. Don't hesitate. Practice instituting these cutbacks right away.

Learning to go to your battle stations the moment weight rises is vital— so expect it to happen and go to work. Continue cutting back until your weight falls into your target zone (about two pounds below Scream Weight), then resume your regular eating plan. Remember that these "reversal days" are an important and unavoidable part of your maintenance life, so find a way to enjoy them. A few days of reversal here and there should be easy for a diet pro like you. For certain, these isolated cutbacks are more pleasant than trying to lose 20, 30, or 100 pounds all over again. You will find that if you allow your weight to creep up over Scream Weight, it will become progressively more difficult to bring it back down. Small fluctuations are probably related to fluid and glycogen, but larger numbers on the scale indicate that fat is coming back. Nip these regains in the bud.

Over time you will become very savvy about the subtle changes in food intake that cause you to gain weight. You will know before you step on the scale whether you are close to Scream Weight. Through practice, lots of practice, you will learn how to control your weight within the target zone without giving it too much thought.

Reversal days should be pleasant and do-able. Make sure you have a prearranged plan to get weight off so that you don't have to wing it at the last moment. The easiest reversal strategy is simply to go back on your original weight loss regimen for a day or two. Obviously, that plan worked for you in the past. Here are some other ideas:

- Try exchanging a diet shake or skim milk coffee product (such as a latte or non-sugar mocha) for breakfast and for lunch. Snack on some fruit or a salad in the mid-afternoon and eat a dinner of lean protein, vegetables, and salad.
- Move your evening meal to lunch and have a light snack instead of dinner. Exercise in the evening.
- Have a diet shake, skim milk coffee product, or fruit smoothie for breakfast. Have fruit and yogurt or soup and salad for lunch and choose a diet frozen dinner (like Lean Cuisine, Weight Watchers, or Healthy Choice) plus a salad for dinner. Do not eat the S Foods (pasta, rice, potatoes) contained in the frozen dinners, however. Substitute some vegetables instead.

Experiment and you will find the plan that works for you. Most important, spend some time cultivating a sense of enjoyment about these reversal days. It's initially annoying to periodically cut back, but in practice you may come to enjoy a feeling of lightness and pleasure when you do.

You will also be helped by exercising a bit more on days that you are reversing. Lowering food intake and ramping up muscle activity puts your body right into fat burning mode—just where you want it to be.

Rule 4 in a nutshell
- Use your Scream Weight to tell you when it's time to reverse your weight.
- Accept frequent reversal days as a fact of life and come to enjoy them.
- When your weight climbs toward Scream levels, put your reversal plan into action immediately.

How to Be 90 Percent Primarian

Rule 5: Eat Primarian 90 Percent of the Time

In Chapters Five and Six, you learned that your genes are programmed for a certain type of diet. If you have not read these chapters, do so now. Our modern reliance on foods that were not part of our original diet has created obesity and disease. POWs have already shown their sensitivity to these foods by responding with uncontrolled eating and avid fat storage. Modern foods will need to be eliminated if they want to avoid the regain cycle.

Rule 5, Step One:
Choose only primarian foods for the first three months
(The opt out period)

Eat from the following menu: Lean meat, poultry, fish, seafood, eggs, vegetables, fruits, nuts, seeds, berries, and low-fat dairy. Add one acceptable treat daily.

Rule 5, Step Two:
After the first three months: design and manage add-backs, but remain 90 percent Primarian

Once you have finished your three-month opt out period, you should still choose Primarian foods almost all of the time. At this point, if you feel that your diet is too restricted, begin a considered program of adding back. But be cautious! Remember: in choosing to dabble with modern foods and S Foods you are headed for a confrontation with your triggers, the foods that addicted you prior to your weight loss. Handle with care. The following guidelines for safely adding back may help:

• **Proceed slowly.**

You will have to figure out how many S Foods your body will tolerate. You are particularly vulnerable to restarting the regain cycle if you previously had Struggling Insulin Syndrome or were addicted to S Foods, so add back one element at a time and watch the scale.

• **Make sure you're in control before you add back.**

Don't begin adding back until you feel that you have established reasonable control over your eating choices. Wait until you are feeling nicely satisfied as an ancient eater. If you're not there yet, continue to eat Primarian and hold off for a bit before playing with add-backs.

• **Limit add-backs to foods from the earth.**

Choose mostly grains, cereals, beans and an occasional sweet potato for adding back as opposed to more modern foods. Continue to practice almost total avoidance of altered foods (things that come in packages and have a complicated list of ingredients). Whole foods are infinitely better choices for adding back than sweets, cakes and things made with white flour.

• **Keep portion sizes small.**

If you decide to add back, a good basic guideline is to start with one modest (half-size) serving daily, and increase or decrease in accordance with your scale response. This may take the form of whole oats for breakfast, a slice of whole grain bread, a controlled portion of a cooked grain, or a half a sweet potato.

• **Use the "is it worth it" test on all other S Foods.**

If you need to make a very occasional departure for a special treat, don't throw it away on gooey white rice, run-of-the-mill bread or soggy fries. If you must choose a modern food—make sure it's something worth paying the price for. Before eating, take a moment to ask yourself, "Is this really that good?" If the answer is yes, go ahead and eat a half portion.

Some Warnings!

• **Don't play with foods that come in little bites.**

Popcorn, chips, small candies, and reduced calorie cookie packs are dangerous. The individual pieces may be small, but these are still addictive S Foods. Remember, there is a reason that the slogan "bet you can't eat just one" had such a ring of truth.

• **Be extremely careful with bread.**

Bread is one of those things that is very hard to stop eating. Remember that bagels, wraps, rolls, and crackers are all forms of bread. If you reintroduce bread, look for the most authentically whole-grain varieties available. Labels should say that the bread is 100 percent whole grain and should list whole-wheat flour as the first ingredient. The fiber content of the bread should equal 2 grams per ounce or more. I suggest that bread be eaten as a single slice only. Try not to return to the habit of eating multiple rolls before a restaurant dinner or of making everything into a sandwich.

• Don't eat salty snacks.

Most snacks combine S elements, like corn, potato, or wheat flour, with salt. We eat vastly too much salt as it is, but both elements in this combination (the salt and the carbohydrate) encourage fluid retention and high blood pressure. Salt is also hard to stop eating.

• Don't be seduced by food labels.

There is a difference between Primarian food and food labeled "organic," "natural," or "unprocessed." Honey is a good example. It can be organic, natural, and unprocessed, but it is still a source of sugar. As a Primarian, remember that your definition of healthy may differ from the one stamped on products by manufacturers. All sources of sugar are to be treated with utmost caution, whether they come from grains, honey, or other naturally grown products. Rely on the list of allowed foods to make your choices. Avoid being swayed by the labels and health claims on foods.

Rule 5 in a nutshell

- Use your knowledge of Primarian diet to choose ancient foods 100 percent of the time in the first three months of maintenance and the great majority of the time thereafter.
- Feel free to add back whole grain products and legumes in small amounts if you wish, but continue to be very wary of other sweets and starches and of packaged foods.
- Carry the Refuse to Regain wallet card (see Resources at the back of this book) for easy reference. When you do make a choice to depart from the plan, make sure it is absolutely worth it and have a small amount only.

Rule 6: Eat One Major Meal per Day

While I don't advise counting calories, the amount of calories you eat after weight loss remains important. To maintain successfully, you will need to match your intake to the smaller demands of your new size. The easiest way to do this is to follow the one major meal rule. Focusing on one complete meal does not mean that you can't eat at other times. In fact, it's important that you do. Your daily plan will have several components:

- One major meal
- Mini-meals

• Meal replacements (optional)
• Fast grabs

Let's define terms. A "major meal" is one that you sit down with, spend a significant time eating, and is composed of a number of different types of foods. In other words, the major meal looks like any typically familiar meal. It might contain a protein source (fish, chicken, meat, eggs), vegetables, fruit, salad, a beverage, and some sort of dessert.

A "mini-meal," on the other hand, is made up of only two foods and substitutes for a regularly scheduled meal. Mini-meal examples are: a can of tuna and a salad, a soup and salad, or low-fat yogurt and some fruit.

"Fast grabs" are smaller snacks which can be added between regular meal times. Grabs should consist of one food only—for example, grapes, mini-carrots, turkey slices, and unsalted nuts. They are eaten on the run. Grab them, don't linger over them—then get out of the kitchen or other food environment.

Your one major meal

You may choose to eat your major meal as your breakfast, lunch or dinner. Feel free to switch the timing as you like. However, once you have decided which meal will be major, plan to eat mini-meals or fast grabs (see below) at other times.

I want to give you some ideas about the look of your major meal. Since you are removing starches from your plate, you may feel you are left with a large hole. All that you really need to do, however, is change your thinking about how a plate should look. Adding fruit to your meal as sauce, salsa, or slices fills up the empty starch area on your plate and adds a new taste dimension. Use many colors, overlap areas, and mix sauces and salsas. Eat large amounts of fiber-containing vegetables. Think about eating without borders—allowing all flavors to mix. Also remember the simple technique of eating by plate pattern: one quarter of the plate protein, three quarters plant foods and a large bowl of greens and salad on the side.

Have as much of everything as you like. Have seconds if you're still hungry. Have fruit for dessert or no dessert (or eat your acceptable treat—you'll read more of this in Rule 10). That's it. This meal works perfectly well whether you are at home or out to eat.

In a restaurant, simply order a piece of chicken, fish, lean meat or other protein. Ask for a double serving of vegetables instead of the obligatory rice or potatoes. Have a salad on the side. Stick to preparations that are simple but flavorful, avoiding frying, breading, and any sauces that sound suspiciously creamy.

Mini-Meals

Sit down and enjoy smaller mini-meals at your two remaining meal times. Remember, the definition of a mini-meal is that it is modest in size and generally contains two elements. If you add more than two components, be very careful to keep the meal controlled in size. Soups and salads are great mini-meals. The heat of the soup makes you feel full and so does the volume. When choosing soups, avoid anything with cheese or cream in its name. Also be careful to avoid the S Foods within, like noodles, dumplings, and matzo balls!

To substitute for some mini-meals, you may want to consider the use of a "meal replacement." Meal replacements are often prepackaged shakes that contain enhanced quantities of vitamins and minerals and are sometimes used for weight loss. I particularly like OPTIFAST® which is a product that was pioneered in Cleveland and which I have been using for weight reduction and maintenance for many years. If you would like to use OPTIFAST®, you will have to hook up with a local program where they can monitor your maintenance and provide the product. (See Resources.) There are other liquid supplements available through health food stores, in pharmacies, and by online purchase. Be careful not to confuse diet meal replacements (usually around 150 calories) with liquids designed to encourage weight gain, such as Boost and Ensure (closer to 250 calories each).

Using a meal replacement once a day reduces choice and decreases exposure to the stimulus of eating. Because the replacement contains a known number of calories, its use assures that energy intake is kept constant. Research into the continued use of meal replacements in maintenance shows that they work to keep weight down. If you prefer, you can design your own form of meal replacement by making breakfast a skim milk coffee product (like a sugar-free mocha or latte), or by designing a fruit smoothie made with low sugar and low-fat components as a substitute for a mini-meal. (See a sample in the Recipe section.)

I generally do not recommend the use of nutritional bars as meal replacements. Most of the commercially available bars look and taste like candy—and seem to have the same effect on the appetite. However, if you can find a bar that works for you and does not make you hungry, it may be a reasonable alternative.

Fast grabs

Fast grabs are healthy, single-food snacks that you can eat on the run throughout the day. I call them "grabs" because I want you to get the idea that these are taken by the handful and are eaten while you are on the move. Do not sit down with snacks and eat them as you would a meal.

You can create your own fast grabs of course, but here are some suggestions: unsalted nuts (but not peanuts, which are actually legumes), grapes, berries, cherry tomatoes, pre-washed carrots, dried fruit (no sugar or high fructose corn syrup added), slices of red, yellow, and green pepper, green beans. Although fast grabs can be eaten throughout the day, please note that we don't need to eat constantly. I suggest giving your body at least two consecutive hours each day during which you don't eat at all. This rest period will give your body a chance to reset its insulin and fat storage mechanisms.

One tremendous help for maintainers is a simple tool my patients call a "readi-pack.". A readi-pack is simply a soft-sided insulated container that travels with you throughout the day. Filled with allowable Primarian foods, your pack gives you an instant supply of good choices and can get you over many tough food moments. (To get an idea of what one maintainer carries, see Carla's section in Chapter Thirteen.)

Eat as many fast grabs as you like as long as you are staying within your goal weight range. If you find that you are gaining weight, look to your snacks first. Common culprits are nuts (healthy, but high in calories), dried fruit (ditto) and salt. Cut back, change spicing, and mix up your snack selection.

Using frozen diet entrees

Our epidemic of overweight has generated a market for low calorie foods. For those who seek convenience, frozen diet meals remain a decent available choice. Brands like Healthy Choice, Lean Cuisine, Weight Watchers, and others offer easily prepared entrees of known calorie content. Generally, they weigh in at between 150 and 350 calories. Frozen entrees can work in your program for several reasons. First, they require little preparation time and decrease your exposure to food. Second, they are quickly cooked, which decreases pre-meal snacking. Third, they can be kept on hand in your freezer as default choices when you've run out of your staple items.

Choose frozen entrees that do not contain S elements like pasta, rice, or potatoes (tough to find). You can use a frozen entrée as either a mini-meal or major meal. If you are using one as a mini-meal, have the entrée alone with a non-caloric beverage. To convert to a major meal, add salad, fruit, additional vegetables, and perhaps a light dessert.

A word about the "breakfast thing"

Conventional wisdom holds that breakfast is the most important meal of the day. The jury is still out on this one as far as I'm concerned. Each of us appears to be different in regard to the timing of our food needs. As a result, the issue of breakfast does not lend itself to one simple rule. Data from the National Weight Control Registry says that successful maintainers eat breakfast. But what does that breakfast look like?

I advise eating a breakfast that fits your hunger level. Most of my patients tell me that they tend not to be particularly hungry in the morning. If you are like they are, the best strategy may be to have something—but not a lot. Skipping food totally does appear to increase hunger later in the day. Worse than forgoing breakfast entirely may be eating cereals, breads, jams and other S Foods that can cause extreme hunger for POWs by mid-morning.

Breakfast is a good time for one of the meal replacements or shakes mentioned above. If you prefer solid food, choosing eggs, fruit, lean poultry, fish, and vegetables in small amounts will work better than the traditional breakfast fare. Hot drinks such as coffee and tea make the stomach feel more full and can be helpful at the start of the day.

Rule 6 in a nutshell
- Eat one major meal per day and mini-meals at the other two meal times.
- Eat fast grabs for energy but clear at least two hours daily for an empty stomach.
- Keep all food choices within ancient guidelines.

Rule 7: Perform a Daily "Scan and Plan"

Each day of weight maintenance is an obstacle course with hurdles that you'll need to clear. Like a trained athlete, you can actually enjoy running the course if you figure out beforehand where the jumps and jogs are likely to occur. To do this, start each day with a Scan and Plan. Before launching into your schedule, think ahead and imagine where and when food is likely to enter your day. (Try doing it during your morning shower.) You'll find that it's easy and surprisingly effective.

You already know what is on your schedule. Maybe you are planning dinner out with friends, meeting a friend at a local coffee bar, and anticipating the challenge of "doughnut day" at work. Briefly envision the day as a whole (the "Scan") and answer the following:

- Which meal will be my one major meal?
- How will I stay Primarian today?
- Will I need to carry food with me?
- Is food assault, secondhand food or sabotage likely? If so, what is my plan for defusing the situation?

Here's what a typical Scan and Plan might look like:

Your scan

Doughnuts at workplace this morning, lunch with client at local restaurant, afternoon meeting (cookies and sodas always present), quick coffee with friend who has been a bit jealous of your weight loss, dinner at home, favorite program on TV...rest of the family will be wolfing down popcorn.

Your plan

Major meal: Dinner with family

Hurdles:

Doughnut day–Take a readi-pack to work with grapes, mini carrots, cherry tomatoes, and unsalted nuts. Mix a diet shake with ice, chunks of frozen fruit, and diet soda. Place in a large container and sip throughout the morning. Physically avoid doughnut room.

Lunch with client–Has to be a mini-meal because dinner is already assigned. Have a large bowl of soup, a nice salad, and a diet drink.

Cookie meeting–Bring cup of hot coffee or tea into the meeting and some sugarless mints. Sit with your back to the cookie tray if possible. If you are really feeling proactive, mention that you've recently succeeded in losing a large amount of weight and ask that the cookies be kept away from you.

Coffee with sabotaging friend–Expect her to offer to split a pastry and make several comments about the way you eat and look. Vow to stay unemotional. Prepare a response. ("I'm feeling such increased energy on this Primarian diet. Maybe you should try it," might do.) Brush her comments off lightly and change the subject. Treat yourself to a non-sugar syrup in your coffee like caramel or sugar-free mocha if you want.

TV snacking–Save your acceptable treat for TV time and enjoy your low-fat ice cream, pudding, etc.If your family must eat popcorn, buy it pre-made so you don't have to deal with the persistent smell.

The Scan and Plan technique may seem obvious to you, but it really works. Don't leave yourself to make choices at the last moment. Visualizing what you will do in each situation actually makes that outcome more likely to happen.

Rule 7 in a nutshell
- Scan your food challenges first thing in the morning.
- Make a game plan, then run the plays.

Rule 8: Stop Eating at 8 P.M.

This rule is straightforward. Food is fuel. If your body is going into a resting state as you enter the evening hours, what is the point of fueling it up as if it were heading into a marathon? Late night eating encourages fat storage and is a major problem for POWs. It is nothing more than a habit. Make the decision that eating ends at 8 P.M. Period. Once you have acclimated to this rule, you will find that being pulled away from it by the occasional late night dinner makes you feel awful.

One other observation on the timing of your food intake: since it makes sense to eat when the body is active, you may find that a good maintenance strategy is placing your major meal at lunchtime. Eating earlier in the day puts calories into the system at the time they are most needed for immediate burning. You may find, as I have, that eating a larger lunch, a smaller dinner and combining the two with evening exercise is a winning formula for weight maintenance. You don't need to do this every day, but try it when you can. For some, it works nicely to keep weight stable.

Rule 8 in a nutshell
- Don't eat when your body doesn't need it.

Rule 9: Eat from a Limited Menu

Choice is stimulating. And confusing. Each morning you awake, go to your closet and select a pair of shoes. How many pair do you choose from? Five? Ten? Think of how much tougher it would be if you had the choice of every pair in the Nordstrom shoe department. Getting dressed would take much longer and would be a lot more anxiety provoking.

In his book, *The Paradox of Choice*, Swathmore professor Barry Schwartz writes that choosing from too many options can be overwhelming, and can even lead to depression. The array of goods available to us can be literally staggering. We find ourselves in the same situation with food.

Perhaps you'd like to take a guess at the number of food products available in today's supermarket. Since 1980, the average number of items on the shelves has more than tripled, increasing from 15,000 to 50,000. That's 50,000 choices for you to contend with. Besides making us anxious, food choice makes us hungrier. A British study had subjects eat as much as they wanted of either five, ten, or fifteen different types of foods. Those subjects with greater choice ate as much as 25 percent more than the others. Other research confirms that menu variety encourages us to eat more. You have undoubtedly experienced this phenomenon yourself when, after feeling stuffed from a large meal, you could still find room for dessert. This is a function of the variety in your food.

Dietary research also supports the technique of "stimulus narrowing" for achieving weight loss. Translated into simple terms, stimulus narrowing simply means cutting way back on food choice. Diets often accomplish this through the repetitive use of meal replacements (shakes, bars, etc.) or meals of similar content. Stimulus narrowing is a very effective tool for weight maintenance as well. All we need to do is give ourselves fewer choices.

What about nutritional content? Don't we have to eat from a wide variety of foods in order to stay healthy? You might believe so. Ancient peoples, however, managed to stay healthy while eating quite limited diets. The Masai in Africa ate a diet consisting of only meat, milk, and animal blood, yet avoided modern diseases. The same is true of the Inuit, who ate primarily blubber, fish, and meat. Today, such restricted menus are no longer necessary. We are lucky to be able to buy fresh fruit in the winter and produce from all over the world year round. This, however, does not mean we can't keep our diets simple.

Principles of eating from a limited menu:

Follow a Primarian diet—Simply by sticking with a hunter-gatherer diet, you will eliminate most overly stimulating food choices. At the same time, you will eat foods of the densest nutritional value.

Pick certain meals as your staples and rotate them or repeat them in your day-to-day plan—You can deviate from these staple meals when you go out or socialize as long as you stay within the general format of the The 12 Tough Rules. On most days, though, know the meals that tend to keep you at goal and repeat a small number of them consistently.

Attempt to stay satisfied with a somewhat plain array of foods—You will know that you are doing this correctly when you feel perfectly fine with what you eat, but are not particularly hungry or interested in lots of other types of foods.

In short, to avoid the pitfalls of overstimulation, stay with meals composed of limited foods most of the time. Construct several meals that are built of permissible foods and which you enjoy eating. Choose these base meals often, varying the components slightly.

Possible base meals:
- Grilled turkey burgers, fresh salsa, sliced fruit or berries, large salad, and cooked broccoli.
- Water packed tuna, sliced avocado, large salad, cooked carrots, and applesauce.
- Lean beef, sliced pears, green beans, cherry tomatoes, and a large salad
- Grilled or poached salmon, mixed vegetables, fruit salsa, and a large salad.

Rule 9 in a nutshell
- Get familiar with a number of healthful meals and snacks.
- Don't get too fancy. Keep food simple most of the time.

Rule 10: Have One Acceptable Treat per Day

In today's food culture, eating serves as a drug, a diversion and a reward. Although our bodies do best with a Primarian diet, we all know that we are no longer-hunter gatherers living in a tribal world. Life's stresses and the constant presence of food make it near impossible to avoid some degree of comfort eating. Rule 10 allows you to indulge, at least partially, your desire to "thrill eat," in other words, eat for pure pleasure.

Schedule one acceptable treat into each day. What makes a treat "acceptable"? It should have these characteristics:

- Delicious enough to look forward to daily.
- Low in saturated fats, no trans fats and not intensely sweet.
- Calorie count totals less than 150 per serving.
- Eating does not stimulate your appetite for more of the same or for other modern foods (in other words, it is not a "gong" food).

If you find that eating your treat causes you to get hungrier or to crave more of the same type of food the next day, abandon that particular choice and find another. Examples of treats that may work for you include things like low-fat frozen yogurts and ice creams, low-fat or sugar-free puddings, and diet ice cream bars, sandwiches, or cones. Many of these foods come in versions made with artificial sweeteners. Choosing these allows you to eat larger servings while staying under your calorie cap. Many of my patients like to top their treat with non-fat whipped toppings.

Once you have selected your treat, find a time of day to indulge in it and savor it. For most, this seems to be in the evening while watching TV. Make sure treat time occurs before the 8 P.M. deadline and pay close attention to the fact that you are learning the new skill of eating a single treat rather than snacking continually throughout the evening hours.

Rule 10 in a nutshell
- Plan on one treat each day.
- Make sure it's not a "gong" food (not excessively sweet or over stimulating).
- Keep the calories at around 150.

Rule 11: Have a Love Affair with Exercise

Exercise is crucial for weight maintenance. At your new lower weight your body is more efficient and needs fewer calories to run. That means you will need to eat quite a bit less than you might want to—unless you burn off calories in another way. Exercise will keep your muscles active and toned, important since muscles are calorie-burning factories. Exercise will maintain your body in a tuned-up state that allows for proper fuel combustion. Exercise insures that your muscles use glucose and insulin in the most effective way. Exercise will enable you to eat more here and there and not pay a price. Recent research even suggests that exercise may lengthen life by keeping chromosomes from aging as quickly as those of the sedentary.

We talk, talk, talk about what to eat, how much to eat, and how to add to, subtract from, and modify our diet. Then we often give ourselves a pass where exercise is concerned. Please don't make this mistake. Although there is much less written in this book about physical activity than about diet, I'm here to tell you that they have equal importance in your warrior's battle with weight regain.

When people are dieting, they often notice that they lose weight whether they exercise or not. As a result, many POWs don't really see the point of lots of exercise. If you are one of these people, now is the time to think again. Exercise assumes a much greater importance in maintenance. You're unlikely to maintain your weight loss without it.

The National Weight Control Registry reports that their average successful maintainer walks four miles per day. That's a significant amount of physical activity. Most of what we hear suggests we simply walk a bit further when we park our car or add small bouts of exercise a few times a day. These are moderation strategies. In the real world, we see successful maintainers doing something quite different.

Since I am about to tell you to get seriously physical, I advise you to follow the familiar advice of seeing your doctor before you begin. This check-up is particularly important for POWs. The burden of past weight may have taken a toll on your cardiovascular system, particularly if you suffered from high blood pressure, elevated blood sugar or high lipids when you were heavier. Even if everything appears to be just fine, it is prudent to start slowly and work up to higher levels of activity.

Here's what you're ultimately shooting for:

- An hour of aerobic activity five to six days per week. (Exercise vigorously, as long as that is safe for you.)
- Fifteen to twenty minutes of weight training on two or three of those days. Weight training can substitute for part of the aerobic work-out so that each exercise bout stays at an hour.

As most of you already know, aerobic activity is the kind of exercise that is continuous—things like dancing, biking, running, or walking fast.

A muscle building activity that uses weights or machines is intermittent and is called anaerobic exercise.

Learning how to exercise correctly is imperative but is beyond the scope of this book. If you'd like to do anything more complicated than vigorous walking, seek some guidance. The least expensive alternative is to seek advice from someone who's already good at your chosen activity.

Novice weight lifters, in particular, should be careful. The potential for injury from poor technique is real. To learn how to lift weights, inquire at a community center, "Y," or gym. Several sessions with a trainer may seem costly but will help you avoid injury over the long-term and will teach you how to get the benefit you want from your workout. Ask whether you can set up a basic training program and continue on by yourself from there. Many trainers will be agreeable. Intermittent follow-ups can advance or adjust your program as you get stronger.

If trainers are beyond your budget, try checking out one of the many videos available in your library to teach you the correct form and procedure for both weight training and aerobic activity.

Getting started is a big step in the right direction, but just lacing up the sneakers isn't enough. The key to making Rule 11 work is developing the love affair it mentions. If you can't imagine ever feeling passionate about the physical it's probably because you've been conditioned to see exercise negatively. In the past you probably:

- Felt sluggish and avoided exertion.
- Associated exercise with boring, painful, repetitive activities.
- Did not see yourself as a coordinated or physical person.
- Hated sweating.

But now is not then. So let's look at this in a new way. Before you settle for an "Okay, I'll force myself" relationship with exercise, try falling flat-out in love with it. Assuming that you are able to exercise without limits, here are my suggestions for finding true love:

Rule 11, Step One:
Make this conscious decision: "I am going to become an athlete."

I know this may sound impossible to you (some of my patients even laugh the first time I say this), but allow the idea to percolate. I define an "athlete" as someone who consistently enjoys a physical activity. Passion and interest are important. Skill level is not.

Developing an athletic identity means that you pursue your sport or activity seriously, that you learn about it, practice it and outfit yourself for it. It also means that others identify you as someone who exercises. Once you have become established in the minds of friends and relatives as a person who is consistently active, that part of your identity will become a valued part of you as well. Even if you see yourself as utterly uncoordinated, there is some sport or activity you can do. Commit yourself to finding it.

Rule 11, Step Two:
Pick a unique sport or activity to fall in love with.

It's easier to be passionate about something thrilling than about something that bores you to tears, so your next job is to discover an exercise that intrigues you. Once you choose, you will need to be persistent. In the beginning, you and your activity will be uncomfortable strangers, kind of an arranged marriage. But remember, love can blossom in time. This may mean spending many months as the clumsy person in the back of a Zumba class or flailing at a ball with a racquet that doesn't want to connect. Stick to it. You'll soon find that the awkward journey to improvement is strangely fun.

What to choose? While walking is the easiest activity to start, it doesn't have to be your first thought. There are some significant problems with walking, including rainy days, winters and lack of partners. While some people find it meditative, others are bored. Walking is a fine choice, but don't pick it because it's the easiest choice. Only choose it if you really enjoy the stroll. The same can be said for ellipticals, stair steppers, rowers, and stationary bikes.

Most of the people I treat do reasonably well on home machines as long as they are actively trying to lose weight. This type of exercise becomes boring once they enter the long haul of maintenance. If solitary machine work-outs make you feel like a hamster on a wheel, don't get started with them. The treadmill is not the only work-out ever invented.

Before you default to a walking program or try to warm up to a soulless machine, take your time investigating other forms of exercise. Go for the bold. Make use of the free trial classes offered by many gyms and studios to try everything from kickboxing to Jazzer-

Some Sports to Choose From

• Aerobics	• Ballroom Dance	• Basketball
• Bowling	• Boxing	• Competitive Frisbee
• Curling	• Fencing	• Folk Dancing
• Hiking	• IceHockey	• Martial Arts
• Racquet Ball	• Skateboarding	• Skating
• Skiing	• Snowboarding	• Snowshoing
• Soccer	• Softball	• Spinning (indoor biking)
• Squash	• Surfing	• Tap Dance
• Tennis	• Volleyball	

cise. Think about sports you've always wished you could play. Take a couple of introductory lessons. Get a little taste of each, then narrow down the field.

Find an activity you can do in a group, small or large. Being involved with others allows you to establish an athletic identity more quickly. In the long run there is an even greater benefit: the people you meet will keep you involved.

Your chosen sport or activity should be one that piques your interest, not one that you are necessarily good at. Remember that your goal is to gradually become skilled. The level at which you begin is completely unimportant. Here are a few possibilities:

Limited in Your Routine?

What if you are too physically limited to exercise? It is still imperative that you burn off some of your daily calories in a way that is deeply satisfying. Types of activity that may involve less strenuous exertion include:

- various forms of yoga
- tai chi
- walking and walking tapes
- water aerobics
- chair based exercise
- light stationary biking
- weighted exercise that avoids areas that are a problem for you

Your chosen sport may or may not lend itself to daily participation. If you have chosen something that can only be done occasionally (tennis, golf, outdoor biking) you will need an alternative activity for off days. Choose something that helps you perform better in your primary activity. This may be the spot for the treadmill or elliptical.

Rule 11, Step Three:
Outfit yourself

Whether it's walking, tennis, yoga, or karate, equipment makes you feel like you belong. Part of your new athletic identity is figuring out which sneakers work best for you, and having the right hat, bat, racquet, or club. Enjoy the process. Equipment does not have to be expensive. Big box stores carry everything from workout suits to yoga mats and there are online options ranging from outlets to eBay. Remember, too, that equipment is an investment in health—one that will pay off big in the future.

Rule 11, Step Four:
Get a goal

All athletes need training goals, and you're an athlete, remember? If your sport is running, your first goal may be to make it through a one minute jog. At the same time, you may want to set a long-term goal of running two miles per day at the end of one year. The person who's chosen aerobics may have the simple goal of moving from the back row of the class to the front as time goes on. Walkers may train to walk a 5K or charity walk at some future time. Bikers have endless opportunities to join yearly group rides. Train for a specific event. Whatever sport you choose, work at it and establish a goal. When that goal is met, celebrate and go on.

Rule 11, Step Five:
Pursue your sport vigorously

While it is true that some exercise is better than none, vigorous exercise is the kind that addicts people. We have talked quite a bit about the harmful addictions imposed on our bodies by modern foods. Here is your opportunity to substitute a craving that will entirely change your life for the better: but only if you work through your beginner's discomfort. The exercise high that you've heard about is very real and awaits you at more advanced levels of performance. Go for it!

Rule 11, Step Six:
Schedule it

You may notice that people who are true exercise fans are generally involved with other athletes. They run in groups, bike together on the weekends, play tennis, or belong to a softball league. Whatever activity you choose, I advise that you, too, link your exercise to others by joining classes or small groups.

One reason to recommend group activity is that it requires you to be responsible to others. Anyone who has ever vowed to use their home treadmill knows that the resolution to workout falls to the bottom of the list by the end of the day. Without a scheduled commitment, exercise doesn't get done.

In the beginning, forcing yourself to exercise is a bit like going to the dentist. Would you show up if there were no appointment and no office full of people waiting for you to appear?

Each week, enter your scheduled exercise times directly into your day planner. Assure that you follow through by committing yourself to group activities, trainers, or partners who, like your dental team, will be unhappy if you stand them up.

Rule 11, Step Seven:
Re-evaluate in two to three months

Even if you are still uncoordinated and clumsy, you should be able to tell within a short time if your chosen sport is worth pursuing. Re-evaluate after several months. Has your activity become drudgery? By all means, ditch it and switch to another. Still intrigued? Continue on no matter how poorly you think you're doing.

Don't expect instant passion. Remember the arranged marriage? You and your sport are two very different entities who just happened to find themselves thrown together. Spend time with each other. Learn about each other. Fail and triumph together. Before you know it, love will bloom.

Rule 11, Step Eight:
Change it up

Try to keep your activity fresh. If you use videotapes, borrow new ones frequently from the local library. Incorporate music that is meaningful to you to deepen the experience.

Follow the steps above that discuss outfitting, goal setting and scheduling. These will be important for you as well.

Slower forms of activity lend themselves to meditation. Practice using your walking, yoga, or slow biking as a time to reflect on your life, to be quiet, and to create an island of pure pleasure in your day. Once again, the key to staying physical is to find a great enjoyment in its practice.

Symptoms of being in love

How will you know when you have fallen hard (in more than a way that skins your knee)? Keep your eye out for the following signs. They will tell you that your relationship with exercise is no longer simply platonic:

- You get annoyed when your exercise class is cancelled or you can't make it.
- You find yourself gazing longingly at athletic equipment on the internet.
- You lose track of time while pursuing your sport.
- You feel better after your sport than before it.
- You experience your first exercise high.
- You revel in the feeling of a good sweat.

Is it possible that you, the person who never wanted to perspire, might become an athlete? Without doubt! Think of all that you have already done to change your habits and your body. Change is manageable. There is some activity out there that you can enjoy and do well. Don't allow yourself to get caught up in the old expectations you once had for yourself. Go boldly forward and work out.

Rule 11 in a nutshell
- Exercise is crucial for maintainers. Find an activity that seems intriguing and practice it five to six days per week.
- Underscore its importance in your life by scheduling it into each day, outfitting yourself and setting goals to achieve.

Rule 12: Maintain with Support and Support Others

It will be much easier for you to maintain your lost weight if you have a guardian to monitor your progress, catch you when you backslide, and support your continued successes. If you do well at maintaining, you will reach what I call the Senior Level in Maintenance (SLIM) sometime toward the end of your first year.

Remain in a supported setting until you feel confident that you have achieved this Senior status. Even better, remain supported permanently. One of my most successful maintenance patients comes to see me once every month. Although she is in perfect control about five years into a 100-pound weight loss, she says that she intends to keep in contact indefinitely.

Where can you find support? Here are some possibilities:

• Meet with a dietician at least monthly.

Explain your maintenance diet and that your goal is to stay below Scream Weight. He or she may help you by having you keep food records or simply by monitoring the foods that may be causing you problems. Be sure that your dietician can support your Primarian eating plan.

• Find an inexpensive weight loss support group.

These can often be found through school districts, community centers, and newspaper sections announcing local events. Weight Watchers groups may work for this purpose. Weigh in at least monthly, more frequently if it is helpful. You will quickly become the star of the show if you are successfully nailing maintenance. Develop relationships within the group, mentor others, and rely on their encouragement.

• Buddy up with friends who are trying to stay at a healthy weight. If no one you know is in this category, you may also partner with people who are trying to lose weight. Whether you are maintaining or losing, there are some basic similarities: sticking to plan, staying committed, and keeping a focus on your goals.

• Ask to weigh-in and meet with a counselor at one of the commercial weight loss programs.

Explain that you are not trying to lose further weight and negotiate a reduced price for this service. Again, insist on following your own plan, not one they impose on you.

- **Start your own maintainer's group.**

There are endless numbers of people just like you who have lost weight and are struggling to avoid regain—they just don't know one another. Try putting an ad in the community announcements section of your newspaper (often run for free) and recruit other warriors like yourself. Invite lecturers, read books on nutritional topics, schedule group bike rides and hikes, ask a dietician to take you on a supermarket tour—the possibilities are endless. You may want to find a dietician, behaviorist, or doctor to run your group. Or you may choose to alternate responsibility for monthly sessions between group members. Weigh in at the start of each session. One tip: don't dwell on slip-ups or spend time discussing individual eating habits. Keep it educational and inspirational.

- **Find an online community.**

Lynn Bering is a writer and weight-loss success story. While in the process of losing 168 pounds, Lynn began blogging about her daily journey. Her story can be followed in The Bering Blog, a wonderful read—both compelling and human.

Lynn was touted as an expert dieter in *People Magazine* and on "The Today Show." Once Lynn entered maintenance, however, she recognized that she was in new and uncharted territory. She was smart enough to know that she needed significant support. As she describes it:

> When I started maintenance, I felt like I was floating, unsure what to do. Four women I knew from the Weight Watchers on-line discussion boards were also at goal and so I asked them if they minded if I asked them questions once in awhile. Their response was overwhelmingly yes because they, too, were wondering if they were doing maintenance "right." We started emailing each other in group emails, but that became too cumbersome so we started a discussion board on QuickTopic.com. We have entered more than 1,700 posts in just seven months.
>
> We talk about everything: food, weight gain, weight loss, the emotional issues of gaining a pound (the "oh my god I'm gaining it all back" syndrome), going too far (the "maybe if I just lose one more pound I'll love myself" syndrome), exercise. You name it, we talk about it. Noth-

ing's off limits. It's the most freeing (and educational) relationship I've ever had with a group of women.

Lynn's experience is one that can benefit all Maintenance Juniors. Consider setting up an online discussion board or getting into the e-mail habit with one or two other maintainers. Lynn reports that she and her support group talk many times a day. If you feel that you would benefit from frequent feedback, encouragement, and hand-holding, you are not alone. You will find others online that feel the same way.

Because the Internet has the power to connect people from all over the world, Lynn and I recently launched a support website specifically for maintainers. Both of us write a blog twice-weekly on a topic that is interesting and/or educational. The site also provides links to many other maintenance-friendly areas on the Internet. There is a recipe page, a question and answer forum, and a discussion area that allows you to converse directly with other maintainers. We look forward to having you join our community, so please visit us at refusetoregain. typepad.com.

Plan to stay in a supported environment for a minimum of one year after your successful weight loss. Once you have maintained for awhile, you will have learned a tremendous amount about yourself and your body.

The knowledge that you will accumulate is so important that Rule 12 includes the direction to share it with others. Becoming a mentor to those who are struggling with their own weight allows you to take a final step beyond just maintaining. It allows you to become the expert. Share your knowledge and experiences with those who seek you out. You can read more about how to do this in the chapter that follows.

You have arrived. It's now time for your efforts to be celebrated and respected. Mentoring others will not only vastly impact their lives, but will enrich your own by providing you with the ongoing reward you truly deserve.

Rule 12 in a nutshell
- Expect to need support and help throughout maintenance.
- Seek out help from professionals or peers.
- Solidify your own maintenance experience by helping others who are trying to lose or maintain weight.

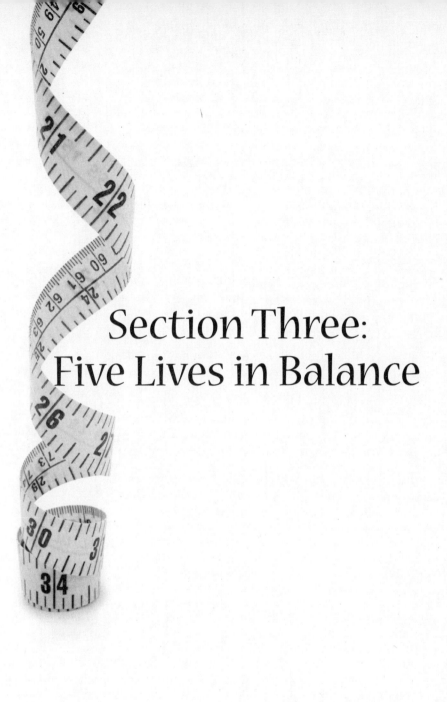

Section Three:
Five Lives in Balance

Chapter Twelve

Junior, Senior, Mentor

Whoever knocks persistently, ends by entering.
　　　　　　—Ali (A.D. 600-661) *Maxims of Ali*

SLIM

At some point during the next year, you will advance from Maintenance Junior to Senior Level Maintainer (SLIM). No bells, whistles, or fireworks will accompany this change—yet you will be aware that you are more comfortable with your food choices and a lot better at managing maintenance than you were before. That's when you will know that an important transition has occurred.

Exactly when will this happen? The time period varies from person to person. Be patient. If you remain strong and focused, your persistence will pay off. While the early stages of maintenance may be challenging, your transition to SLIM will bring a sense of greater peace and freedom.

Here are some additional clues to help you know that you've arrived at your destination:

> **Clue:** You rarely miss your old way of eating.
> **Clue:** You enjoy and actually prefer your new eating habits.
> **Clue:** You no longer feel controlled by food.
> **Clue:** You are comfortable with eating many of the same types of foods repeatedly.
> **Clue:** You are not particularly interested in S or altered foods.
> **Clue:** When you do occasionally eat these foods, you are not compelled to overeat and are able to return to your plan the next day.
> **Clue:** When you choose to eat foods that are off your plan, you generally find them less enjoyable than you thought you might.

Clue: You know intuitively the foods and amounts that will keep you from gaining weight.

Clue: You are acutely aware of the unhealthy diet habits of those around you.

Big clue: You feel free.

Moving from Junior to SLIM does not mean that you will never miss modern foods nor that this state will last permanently. Even at the most senior level, you may be able to sustain maintenance for a period and then find yourself weakening. This seems to be normal for most maintainers, so don't let it throw you.

What is important is that you identify problems and address them. When weakening occurs, seek help the moment you see that you cannot get things under control. A weekly weigh-in program or a dietician can turn things around.

While SLIM status does not mean that you'll never have a difficult day, it does mean that you have made peace with the way you think about food, physical activity, and priorities. That mental change is huge.

Weight Mentors

Becoming a SLIM is a great accomplishment, but there is a final level of weight maintenance expertise you can reach if you choose. Just above the Seniors are the super-maintainers I call "Weight Mentors." Mentors often become interested in nutrition and in keeping up on its latest developments. They keep in touch with their POW history by drawing on their own experience to counsel those who are struggling.

People you meet during your Junior year may not be aware that you were once heavy. If you are comfortable with sharing this information, go ahead and reveal it. This opens up the the topic. Opportunities to help others will often follow.

Weight Mentors can be found leading weight loss groups, writing about their experiences, becoming personal trainers, and giving talks. Some simply see themselves as active mentors to friends and family. Their coaching skills can be responsible for the weight loss of large numbers of people.

If you have successfully lost weight and are making that loss stick, you possess information and experience that is of extreme value to others. You may think that everyone knows what you know. They don't. I believe that the true obesity experts are those who have vanquished the problem. That's you. So recognize that you have something very real to offer.

To move up to Mentor status, continue to read and learn about food choice, metabolism, and diet. Form your own opinions. Catalogue the books and articles you think are worthwhile. Keep a list of resources and the names of people who helped you on your journey. When someone asks you how you lost weight, offer to meet them over coffee and tell them what you know. Point them in the right direction and share resources. If you want to offer even greater support, check in with them by e-mail, make weekly phone calls or arrange future meetings.

You may want to consider leading a weight-related group, as described in Rule 12.

If you are a parent, how about getting involved in your kid's school? Now that you know how important exercise is, wouldn't it be great to spearhead a movement to get more physical education into your child's day? And what about the lunches at school? If they are largely non-Primarian (full of starch, sugar, and altered foods) you may be able to prevent obesity from getting a foothold by working to change the menu. Does your child's curriculum include a unit on nutrition? Are there vending machines on site and do they still contain full sugar sodas and juices? There are many opportunities to be an activist.

A few other ideas:

- Start a walking group.
- Write to government officials about the importance of developing wellness programs and incentives.
- Convince your town to build bike paths.
- Work to get food out of your workplace by confining eating to mealtimes and to a designated lunchroom or kitchen.

If we are to change the way our country eats and lives, it's going to have to start with a grassroots effort. You can be on the forefront. The ways in which you can affect the lives of others are endless.

A special opportunity to help:
The National Weight Control Registry
If you have lost over thirty pounds and have kept the weight off for one year or more, I urge you to take a giant step toward Mentor status by joining the National Weight Control Registry. I've referenced this

ongoing study throughout previous chapters and you may have the opportunity to be part of it.

The National Weight Control Registry has been collecting data on maintainers since 1994 as a joint project of Brown University and the University of Colorado. It is a "prospective" study. That means that participants will be followed into the future to see what happens to their maintenance efforts. Collecting this information is key. From Juniors and Seniors like you, weight loss professionals can learn what works and what doesn't. They may also find that successful weight maintenance is more common than people think. Documenting this offers hope to all those who dream of being leaner permanently.

Some of my patients are fearful of joining the registry because they don't want to be the one person who fails. *If you have successfully lost weight and are making that loss stick, you possess information and experience that is of extreme value to others.* If this is concerning you, please don't let that worry stop you from participating. Studies learn just as much from slip-ups as they do from perfection and no one in the study is perfect.

I believe that membership in the registry is a badge of honor for those who are trying to permanently control weight. You will receive a yearly questionnaire that asks about your diet, exercise habits, and current weight. Participation can help keep you focused on the importance of daily habits and reinforces that you are a serious maintainer.

For information about joining the National Weight Control Registry, visit their website at nwcr.ws. There is no cost to you, other than your time, but the rewards are great both for you and for science.

Chapter Wrap

- Remaining tough, pushing past the temptations to eat, being consistent—these are the tasks you are struggling with today in your quest for Senior or Mentor status.
- In the next chapter, you will read about five people who have successfully negotiated those struggles. At one time, each one of them stood in your shoes. At one time or another, each lost weight and put it all back on. But finally, things were different. Let their stories stand as proof that you, too, can keep off your weight if only you refuse to regain.

Chapter Thirteen

Five Lives in Balance

Life is like riding a bicycle. To keep your balance you must keep moving.
—Albert Einstein

The five people profiled in this chapter actually exist. I know each of them. Their stories are written just as they told them to me. Just as dieters have their own personal strategies with weight loss, each maintainer finds solutions in his or her own way.

These maintainers' techniques will not fit you exactly. They serve only to provide ideas and inspiration. In the coming months and years, you will discover the small secrets, particular to you, that allow you to walk the maintenance tight rope. Always keep in mind that you are involved in a balancing act—one in which small shifts in direction, a push or a puff of wind can lead to a tumble. What these five maintainers demonstrate is that, if you keep your eyes forward and keep moving, you can and will succeed.

Bonnie: Senior Level Maintainer (SLIM)
She figured it out on her own

As a denizen of our local fitness center, I have gotten to know many avid exercisers. Many of the same faces (and bodies) have frequented the facility for years. Since I am tuned into body size, I find it interesting to watch people diet, shrink, and then balloon up again. This phenomenon seems to occur more frequently in those who are over forty, even if they are very active. Despite being committed exercisers, they seem unable to keep lost weight off for very long.

For this reason I was particularly curious when I saw Bonnie, who is seventy years old, lose an impressive thirty pounds four years ago and keep it off. Bonnie is not my patient. In fact, before this interview we'd never had a discussion about weight at all. Intrigued to find out if she had intuited some version of the 12 Tough Rules, I lured her to a local coffee shop for a chat.

Bonnie, who looks far younger than her age, was in workout clothing when we talked. She exercises five to six days per week quite vigorously. She works out by doing step aerobics and by using a treadmill, a stationary bike, and an elliptical trainer.

"I have a lot more time on my hands now," she said while sipping a coffee with skim milk. "Having the time to exercise has made a big difference. I want to look nice, that's another thing. I also don't want to feel awful." I can vouch for the fact that, having watched Bonnie in aerobics class, she both looks great and is vitally alive.

Bonnie works out both at home and at the fitness center, a practice which has created a strong athletic identity. All of her friends, and many who know her peripherally, think of her as an exerciser.

But how does she manage her eating? I wondered whether she had figured out the secret of Primarian diet on her own.

When I asked Bonnie if she avoided certain food types, she wasn't aware that she did. She believed that she was controlling her maintenance weight with smaller portions. But a bit of closer questioning revealed that, indeed, Bonnie was 90 percent Primarian. At the beginning of her weight maintenance Bonnie had cut out all sugars. After a time, her weight crept up and she realized that sugars had gotten a toe-hold in her diet without her realizing it. She cut them out again, returned to her base weight and did not let them back in her menu. Bonnie does not like cereals or rice and eats no potatoes or desserts, thus eliminating most of the starchy S Foods. She does, however, like bread and has been able to add a small amount back successfully. However, as you will see, she is quite controlled about the amount.

"I love the taste of vegetables now," Bonnie volunteered. She also noted that while she was easily able to control occasional deviations from plan, she no longer had much of a desire to go off course: one of the marks of a true SLIM.

I asked Bonnie to be a little more specific and reconstruct her average daily menu. Interestingly, she told me that she started each day with breakfast—but not until noon. She routinely skips a morning meal because she has never been particularly hungry then. Instead, she opts for eggs, toast, and coffee for lunch. She and her husband often eat dinner out in a restaurant. Bonnie usually chooses fish, accompanied by salad and vegetables.

"I haven't had red meat in a while," she told me. Between meals, hunger is kept at bay with four to five pieces of fruit. You'll notice that, except for the toast with her "late breakfast," Bonnie didn't mention eating any altered or modern foods at all. She also described eating the same types of foods on most days. "The scale doesn't vary that way," she said.

In summary, Bonnie is a successful SLIM who figured out most of the 12 Tough Rules on her own. She eats scarcely and from a limited menu. She may look as if she eats two major meals per day, but because she completely eliminates a morning meal, she is able to keep calories low, a personal adaptation that works well for her. She follows a 90 percent Primarian diet and loves daily exercise. The amount and intensity of exercise is high and she loves what she does. She is tough, not moderate with her program. She also weighs daily and has a plan for immediate reduction when her weight increases. She thinks about what she is eating each day in a way that is very much like a "Scan and Plan." She is making her weight loss work despite the decreases in metabolism that are said to accompany older age. She looks vital and feels terrific.

Grady: Senior Level Maintainer (SLIM)
Working the bank account

Grady is a fifty-year-old attorney whom I've known for twenty years. He was a chubby guy when we first met but always had an interest in athletics, particularly hockey. Grady often talked about the league he played in and about his periodic trips to hockey camps where intense play occurred. Despite his serious interest in skating and his occasional forays into competitive athletics, Grady's overweight state remained unchanged year after year. Sometimes, his frustration with being too heavy would surface during one of our professional meetings. After we'd put aside legal matters, we'd talk about diet. Nevertheless, he remained the same size.

In the spring of 2001, I called Grady for some advice. I hadn't seen him in about a year and he suggested we meet to discuss the matter at hand. We were getting together at my home, so I put on a pot of coffee and bought some store-baked brownies. In general, I don't believe in forcing other people to eat as I do. Grady loved to meet over cake and I always made sure it was available for him.

When I answered the door I was stunned to find a lean, athletic-looking man who bore only a slight resemblance to the person I was expecting. Grady had lost forty pounds. Moreover, he looked as if he'd always been thin. He was clearly delighted by my reaction.

The brownies went uneaten that day, but over coffee, skim milk and sugar substitute, Grady vowed the vow of all dieters: "I'm never going back to the weight I was." Unlike most Juniors, and completely without my help, Grady made good on that promise. He has now maintained his weight for six years with no appreciable period of regain.

Grady experienced an initial weight correction after losing his forty pounds. The 145 pounds he weighed at the end of his diet turned out to be too low to maintain, and he stabilized at around 150. As I mentioned in the discussion on setting Scream Weight, this upward correction often happens to Juniors, particularly those who reduce to very low weights. Once Grady's weight stabilized, he found maintenance to be utterly achievable.

Like Bonnie, Grady is a SLIM who figured out maintenance on his own. Again, I was curious to see how many of the 12 Tough Rules he followed. What I discovered was someone who follows the framework of the Rules, but has been able to add a bit more flexibility than most.

Grady is tough and not moderate. He carefully controls his food intake and weighs himself daily. He also watches how his clothes fit and makes small modifications to his day if he notices any change. He exercises at least six days a week, and often seven by walking for fifty minutes to an hour on a treadmill, supplemented by free weights. He also plays hockey and continues to attend clinics and camps. He is strict in his complete elimination of some foods, particularly fried foods. "Those just don't exist in my universe," he told me. In addition, Grady has served as a mentor to a number of people. "Seeing what I've been able to do has inspired quite a few of the people I work with," he says.

Grady deviates from the 12 Tough Rules, however, by exceeding the 90 percent Primarian rule. He particularly likes bread and the crunch provided by animal crackers. He has not eliminated these foods and even eats a lot of them. About once a month, he will go to his favorite bakery and get treats, usually Russian tea biscuits. "I eat these foods, but I pick my spots," he tells me. In general, he eats more grain-based foods than I would recommend for most maintainers—and he's able to get away with it. Why?

Maintainers are like spenders who have to learn how to operate on a very limited bank account. Most cannot tolerate large amounts of S and altered foods. The type of "spending" that Grady does only works for the limited number of maintainers that have a little more "cash" on hand. These maintainers are:

- Generally, either young or male.
- Very active and able to burn off extra S calories.
- Without manifestations of a weak insulin system prior to weight loss.
- Highly disciplined and organized.
- Without a history of significant S Food addiction prior to weight loss.

Grady's prescription for success works perfectly for him, yet it may not for others. His story illustrates an important point. Maintainers are different. In order to find out where you fall in the spectrum, the best advice is to begin by following the 12 Tough Rules just as they stand. Add the adjustments that work for you only when you are stabilized.

Lois: Endangered Senior Level Maintainer (SLIM)
Hanging on!

Six years ago, Lois lost 150 pounds in our clinic and went from a weight of 313 to a weight of 165. She had lost over 100 pounds two times previously and had regained every ounce quickly. Not this time. For five years, her maintenance was perfect. During that five-year period she completely avoided altered foods and S Foods. She weighed every day and carefully planned out her meals. She ate from a limited menu. She adopted a Primarian approach. She ate one allowable treat a day, a low-calorie ice cream or a fat-free pudding.

Lois's job as head nurse in a busy doctor's practice was often challenging. Drug company representatives brought food into the office daily, and not just any food. The fare usually ran to steaming trays of lasagna, brownies, sodas, ribs, and other tempting treats. Holidays saw a stream of cookie trays, chocolate baskets, cheeses, and goodies. In the beginning, Lois had to remove herself from the fray during lunchtime. She complained to other workers about their eating in her presence, but they refused to change their habits just to suit her. "It bothered me for months," Lois told me, "but after that I got used to it."

Lois was great about sticking to the 12 Tough Rules, even joining the National Weight Control Registry. There were two rules, however, on which she slipped up. First, she never exercised. Second, she didn't establish a Scream Weight or a plan to immediately reverse regain.

After five perfect years of maintenance, Lois regained twenty-five pounds over several months. She still looked terrific (after all she was maintaining a 125 pound loss) but knew that she was in trouble. When I asked her what was causing the problem, she identified it immediately. During a period of family stress, she had begun to allow S Foods back into her diet. At first it was just a taste here and there, but it had gotten out of control. She admitted to eating bags of popcorn and sugary shakes. She was having a bowl of ice cream a night, and it was the high sugar, saturated-fat kind. Bread, potatoes, and rice had strangely also found their way back into her diet.

I asked Lois to describe the foods she had missed when she was in her period of perfect maintenance. She answered that she hadn't missed any, that she had enjoyed eating her particular menu and had never tired of it. When we talked about whether she had ever felt deprived, she paused and then made this poignant observation. "What I miss, what I really miss, is not any of the foods I can't eat. It is eating the way I did then, when I was under control."

Lois's story illustrates the enormous power of S Foods. Remember that POWs will fall out of balance when S Foods reappear in their diet. Insulin appears to re-establish dominance, causing hunger and fat storage. Even those who have achieved Mentor status are vulnerable. No matter how long your experience as a maintainer, your genes and the way they recognize food will not change. If you are a person who has a past history of S Food sensitivity, that characteristic will remain with you. The problem will resurface if you challenge your sensitive system with those foods.

As you know only too well, S Foods have an addictive nature. Once Lois began to "taste," she fell quickly under their spell. Serious food creep ensued. This is the reason, by that way, that I worry about Grady's approach for most maintainers. While he appears able to stave off addiction, most POWs cannot.

Lois and I discussed the importance of adopting an immediate cold turkey attitude toward S Foods. Had Lois been using the Scream Weight rule, she would have had a great deal of practice in small weight reductions by now. She would have learned to cut off S Foods quickly, and would hopefully have remained within close range of her achieved weight.

Lois's lack of exercise also left her without another back up mechanism for disabling food creep. Frequent small reductions work best, achieved by a combination of calorie cutbacks and increased activity.

I'm glad that our scheduled interview for this book gave me the opportunity to hear about Lois's tumble. We will be working together to get her back on track.

Carla: Weight Control Mentor
Taking it two steps further

It's great to see Carla striding toward our meeting place. As always, she is perfectly groomed and carrying a neat stack of folios and books. As it happens, I have brought her clinic chart with me. I quickly check the "before" photo mounted on the inside cover. I'm actually a bit shocked at how overweight Carla was—a bit disheveled and wearing non-descript, over-sized clothing. The Carla who greets me now has glowing skin and a bright smile. No one seeing her would identify her as someone who was once heavy.

Carla is not only a SLIM, she is a Weight Mentor. Throughout her weight loss, Carla was highly interested in learning about the process. She read many articles and books about weight and nutrition, ordering books from distant libraries and online. In fact, her appetite for learning seemed almost to supplant her former appetite for food.

With a background in lifestyle coaching, it seemed perfectly natural for Carla to become interested in helping others in our program. She soon developed a group for patients who were struggling with complex issues surrounding their weight loss. As time went on, Carla also took on patients individually, providing them with much needed education, insights, and mentoring.

Carla, who is in her mid 50s, had lost weight many times in the past and had been on "more diets than you can count." Her successful losses had never exceeded twenty pounds. She'd lost this much on four different occasions, but had never been able to keep the weight off. At our clinic, Carla was able to lose over sixty pounds. When I asked her what made this attempt different, she answered honestly, "Absolute, complete desperation and desolation. I refused to live like that and I said, No more."

Carla's strong feelings were moving—and familiar. Many dieters express this kind of desperation. But it is important to note that it is exactly this intensity of feeling that lets dieters behave in a tough, not moderate, way. The trick is to continue to have this sense of urgency throughout the Junior phases of maintenance, for about a year, until a new diet pattern is set in place.

I asked Carla how often she thinks about what she is eating and she told me that she is "constantly thinking about it." She added wryly, "When I don't is when I get into trouble."

She exercises six days per week. On three days, she has taken up the leadership of a free weight group and teaches other women how to design their own program. This is yet another way in which Carla serves as a Mentor. She decided to take on this role after spending a goodly sum of money on personal training. Once she learned the requisite skills, she realized that she would be able to pass them on to others, at far less cost. In order to stay current, Carla meets with her trainer monthly for a refresher and to advance her own weight program if needed.

On non-free-weight days, Carla does an hour on the treadmill or uses other machines.

Because Carla lost weight in our program, you won't be surprised to hear that she follows Primarian principles. She told me that her biggest challenge is avoiding pasta. "That was my drug of choice," she said. "Before I started this, I would have mainlined it if I could. Now, my extra treat is nuts. But about once a month, my sister comes to town. We go to a restaurant we both really like and share one slice of chocolate cheesecake. That's my big deviation."

I asked Carla if her new way of life made her happy and she said, unequivocally, that it did. She continues to get pleasure each day from remaining at her lower weight. On the other hand she admitted, "I am often tempted severely to eat as I used to. I have to reorient myself each and every day."

Carla uses a Scream Weight to monitor herself and returns to her weight loss plan (three liquid supplements and one meal) when her weight creeps up.

I was curious as to whether she noticed the difference between her own eating patterns and those of her friends. Many of my patients report being horrified by the amount and type of food they see others eating. Carla's answer was a bit different. "Seeing what other people eat makes me feel vulnerable," she said, "so I try to block it out. Sometimes I can eat a whole meal with someone and if you asked me later, I wouldn't be able to tell you a thing they'd eaten."

Because Carla has worked with quite a number of weight management patients, I wanted to know if she had developed any effective aids for maintenance. She immediately produced the following list:

- Having a visual stimulus is very important. I carry a picture of my heavy self in my wallet. I look at it before I go into a restaurant and say, "Never, never again."
- In order to succeed in maintenance, you have to know how to manage irritation, sadness, anger, and fear. If those emotions are throwing you off, seeking counseling or entering a group is important.
- When I feel like eating, I go inside myself and try to put a label on what I'm feeling. Sometimes I'm frustrated or bored. Often a bag of green beans will do just fine—I call this my "green bean test."

Carla's Readi-Pack

Carla insulates her food with freezable ice blankets. These are flexible sheets with individual segments. They fold easily around foods or can be clipped into rows to cool smaller items. See the Resources section for purchasing information.

Carla's packing list:

- Cut up veggies...cucumbers are one of my favorites
- Kosher dill pickles...since I crave salt. (An entire jar is only 65 calories... but I only have 1 or 2.)
- Fruit...grapes keep very well
- Diet shake...always
- Zero calorie diet drinks
- I pack Crystal Light lemonade in my drink containers all summer long and in the winter hot water with lemon slices
- I roll up lettuce leaves: Take a couple and create a solid center of lettuce, then roll a deli slice of low-fat Swiss cheese or turkey or whatever. I get the thinnest slices possible...just for flavor and continue to wrap lettuce until it looks like a super fat Slim Jim. Then roll up in plastic wrap.
- Raw nuts, unsalted

- You've got to find substitutes. For example, for "creamy" I like fat-free ricotta whipped up with calorie-free caramel flavoring. I put it in a beautiful dish, put some fat-free whipped cream on it and eat it with a demitasse spoon.
- Don't leave home without your readi-pack. Fill it with drinks and crunchies. One of my tricks is to take a nutrition bar and cut it up into smaller pieces. I put each piece in a separate bag as a small snack. I also have a host of insulated bags, so I can choose the one that fits my mood for the day. (See the contents of Carla's typical readi-pack in the box on the previous page.)
- I stay away from all of the 100 calorie packs that are out there...they only trigger my hunger.

As you can see, Carla is a highly successful maintainer who still struggles with the alterations she's made to her diet. While some maintainers easily make peace with new eating styles, others simply have a harder time. Carla has helped herself stay balanced by becoming an expert in the very area that has given her trouble. If you are the type of person who likes to teach, lead and inspire, becoming a Weight Mentor will help you to stay in touch with you own goals while truly changing others. Weight Mentoring is a great way to add while subtracting, the strategy described under Tough Rule 2.

Sophie: Weight Mentor

Perfection!

On a frigid January day I met Sophie at a local McDonald's. We talked over bottled water and diet soda as the smell of fried foods, potatoes, and something strongly chemical floated in the air. There was a strange justice in our choice of meeting place. Fast food had lost all power over us. We might as well have been sitting on a park bench.

Looking at Sophie's delicate face and petite bone structure, one would never guess that just four years ago she had weighed 128 pounds more. At only five feet, Sophie had been morbidly obese. Sophie was one of those thin kids who started to gain weight in her teen years. The process accelerated through her twenties. "I never exercised," she said, "but I had an active job and had to do a lot of walking up and down the halls of a large office building. I thought that was enough."

Clearly something was wrong with this thinking, because by the time Sophie was thirty, she was 100 pounds overweight. "I went on a liquid diet and got down to 118 pounds," she said, "but I never learned what to do after that. I tried to exercise, sometimes up to an hour and a half a day, but eventually I just ballooned up and the weight came back." Sophie then became a diet sampler, trying Weight Watchers, the Grapefruit Diet, and a succession of plans she found in magazines. Not a thing appeared to work. Finally, in her late fifties, Sophie came to our private practice for weight reduction.

After a very successful weight loss induced by a combination of OPTI-FAST® supplement and Primarian eating, Sophie nailed her maintenance. In the four years since losing her 128 pounds, she has never exceeded her Scream Weight. In other words, she has maintained perfectly in a range three to five pounds above what she weighed at the end of her diet.

Here are some of the questions I asked Sophie at our meeting, her answers, and my own thoughts:

You have dieted many times and the weight has come back. Was there some special motivation this time?

"This time it was about health. My knees and joints were really bothering me but most of all I got scared about my breathing. I was down to being able to go up and down the steps at home once a day. Then I got sleep apnea and that really frightened me. But even with these motivations, the fear or being sick wouldn't have helped me keep the weight off. It was the education I got about how to eat that made the difference."

Dr. B's comments: *Serious medical complications often motivate excellent weight loss, but the memory of previous illness can fade quickly once the pounds are gone. Following a well thought out plan is key for all maintainers.*

Which maintenance techniques help you most?

"First: the accountability. I am accountable by choice. I come in to be weighed and see you once a month." (Sophie then pulls out a picture of herself, which she keeps in her wallet. It was taken at her niece's wedding when she was at her highest weight. Clearly, this picture helps her to remember who she once was and the place to which she never wants to return.) "I think about what I eat at every meal and I weigh myself daily. I also exercise using videotapes six days a week. I added another tape that has me using three and five pound weights two days a week. I added sit ups and push ups recently too.

"I also plan out what I'm going to eat before the day starts. I eat certain breakfasts on certain days and certain lunches on other days. I change the kind of meat or protein in my dinner every day. I try to eat lots of different colored fruits and vegetables, but I find that I actually eat mostly the same ones. And if I'm going somewhere, I'll plan for it. For example, I attend a Bible study group where they always serve pizza. I just stick an apple in my purse. In fact, I'll always take fruit and my own salad dressings when I go out because I know they'll never have that. Another thing that I do is read a lot about nutrition and diet. I don't read cookbooks, though, because the foods I eat are pretty plain."

Dr. B's comments: *Sophie's answer reveals that she follows most of the 12 Tough Rules including eating from a limited menu, performing a daily Scan and Plan, having an exercise plan she loves, maintaining in a supported environment and being tough, not moderate.*

Are there any foods that you completely exclude?

"Potatoes, rice, pasta, cookies, and cakes (I only take a bite on special occasions). Essentially no processed foods...I don't have any room for these calories with all the fruits and vegetables I eat."

Dr. B's comments: *And, she is 90 percent Primarian.*

Do you keep a food diary?

"No. I used to when I first started out, but now I know pretty much what and how much to eat. I don't count calories or keep any records. I just watch the scale every day to check myself."

Dr. B's comments: *She uses daily weighing and Scream Weight to monitor herself. With practice, she has learned exactly how much to eat to keep her weight controlled. No counting or other monitoring techniques are necessary.*

What do you do to reverse regain if your weight goes up a bit?

"It is very easy for me to gain if I add things. I can go up four pounds on the next day after a family gathering. If this happens, I'll give up my afternoon snack for a few days and my weight will come back down."

Dr. B's comments: *She has established an immediate reversal plan that works for her.*

What are the "treats" in your diet?

"A bite of some special dessert every once in a while. On a daily basis, I love my breakfasts of two poached eggs alternating with oatmeal on the opposite day. Those are some of my only grains. At nine o'clock, my big treat is a half-cup of frozen yogurt. I look forward to my coffee after supper and my three o'clock trail mix and yogurt and cup of tea. I really enjoy that I have sort of set it up in my brain: I get home from work and it's a relaxing time. It's my time."

Dr. B's comments: *Sophie has found a way to incorporate some S Foods like oatmeal and whole grain bread into her plan. But she doesn't pick high sugar foods. The S Foods she's added back are whole foods.*

Do you find the repetition in your diet boring?

"I don't find it boring at all. Too much variety makes it tougher."

Is there an actual enjoyment about what you do?

"Absolutely. I guess I get satisfaction or joy out of that success. I don't get excited so much about the fact that I look better as that I'm succeeding. You know, every day I see other people around me eating whatever they want and I'm eating my carrots. When they're moaning and groaning after they're full, I feel fine. I enjoy it every day."

So you don't ever feel deprived?

"Really, I can't say that I have had any feelings like that. Before, on my other diets, I forced myself not to taste things. When I was on a cruise recently, I tried some desserts and I was fine, so I know I can do special things once in a while. I have my bites."

Dr. B's comments: *Sophie exemplifies the maintainer who has completely changed lifestyle and has come to love the new way she lives. Like someone who is committed to a vegetarian diet or a religiously restricted diet, she would not think of deviating from plan. This is the comfort level that can be achieved by maintainers if they practice their new way of life long enough. It is also what we hope to achieve when we say we want to "change lifestyle." This means not just doing a few things differently, but remaking your way of living and coming to prefer that new way of life.*

On the other hand, Sophie is maintaining perfectly by exerting extreme control over her diet. She still weighs and portions out her food, rarely changes her menu and eats very sparingly. Because she is so controlled, she rarely has to implement reversal days. This method works for her and is the ultimate example of someone who is tough and not moderate. For maintainers who want more flexibility, however, accepting reversal days as a necessary part of life is important. You can be happy with your new life and also accept small "waves" in your weight...as long as you are willing to reverse them quickly.

What kind of maintainer will you be? When you find your way, I hope you will write and tell me your own story. I would particularly like to hear from those of you who have adopted a primarily Primarian lifestyle. How long did the transition take? What supports did you use to keep yourself on course? What wisdoms can you share?

Chapter Fourteen

Six Final Thoughts

It's now time for us to part ways and for you to head off on your maintenance journey on your own. If you've gotten this far, I know you're well-equipped, committed, and capable. I have just a few more thoughts to leave with you.

Seek Harmony

Has it every occurred to you that when you eat, you take a piece of the outside world into yourself? Eating is perhaps the most intimate expression of your reliance on the Earth. You take Earth's products in, internalize them and they become an actual part of you. Only you can define what you choose to become through eating.

Eating is just one way of many ways in which we are interdependent with the larger world. Just as we have departed from ancient dietary patterns, we have also left behind time-honored ways of being part of the natural order. Normally, that order would create a sense of harmony. Many (including myself) believe that the extent of our departure from ancient patterns has been measured in ever-increasing stress and illness.

Nature has designed us to need the sun, for example. Vitamin D is produced through a complex interaction between the sun and your skin. We can live indoors, spend hours under fluorescent lights, and take Vitamin D, but the harmony is gone. We are left with the nagging feeling that we are missing something.

Returning in some degree to our ancient relationship with the Earth is an important adjunct to your new weight and eating plan. This relationship includes: spending more time in the outdoors, enjoying the sun and seasons; working your body; spending quiet time with your own mind; getting to know plants and animals; and having greater respect for natural sleep cycles. I highly recommend each of the above to contribute to a sense of total balance that cannot be provided by diet change alone.

Return to Your Task Calmly

If you have ever meditated, you know that a core principle is concentration on the process of breathing. Meditation teachers will tell you that it is inevitable that your attention will wander. When this happens, you are directed to calmly bring your focus back to the breath.

This is very much the process I suggest you invoke in your first year as a maintainer. I have asked you to focus on the 12 Tough Rules, but your attention to this task is bound to wander. When this happens, your job is to take notice and calmly redirect yourself.

I want to reiterate here that you must spend a significant amount of time living the Primarian life before it becomes preferable to you. So give yourself a chance. Continue to try. And when you do fall off, stray, or otherwise lose your way, see your departure as inevitable, simply part of the process. Don't bother with self-blame or frustration. Calmly redirect yourself and pick up where you left off.

Appreciate Your Success

Although I have laid down what may seem like locked-in-cement rules for weight maintenance, you will ultimately make many modifications. When it comes to something as complex as living, there is no one-size-fits-all.

Success is not a measure of how perfectly you follow my plan, but of how good you are at developing yours. You can count yourself successful if you create a plan, commit to it and are tough in following it.

How much weight must you keep off? Obesity experts frequently emphasize that a loss of 5 percent to 10 percent of your original weight significantly reduces your chances of developing weight related disease. If you are a woman who once weighed 180 pounds and now weighs 144, your thirty-six pound loss represents an impressive 20 percent drop. It would be terrific if you could anchor at this lower weight, but suppose you just can't make that happen?

Remember that keeping off even much smaller amounts will be good for you. If you stabilize at 171—just nine pounds under your original weight— you will be maintaining a 5 percent weight loss. That may not be perfect or exactly what you wanted, but this amount of sustained weight loss is a boon to your health and represents a real accomplishment. Most of America is gaining weight. If you have lost at least 5 percent, and have not returned to what you once weighed, you and your body have a lot to feel good about.

Protect Your Kids

Many of my patients ask about the proper diet for their children. Since your kids carry your genetic traits, it is logical to assume that they will be sensitive to the modern Western diet just as you are. As parents, we are constantly preparing our children for the dangers they may meet. Don't talk to strangers. Don't give in to the friend who offers drugs.

The danger of becoming obese and sick from our Western diet lies squarely in the path of your children. Now is the time to prepare them.

My advice to parents is that you talk to your children about your Primarian eating style and model the importance of health. Show your children that you are strongly committed to keeping yourself in good shape and at a healthy weight.

Keep things largely Primarian within your four walls and put a strong limit on modern treats for your children. You will not be able to control what your children eat outside the home, despite everything that you are led to believe. They will get plenty of access to junk foods and modern sweets elsewhere. Other than reminding kids about your beliefs, I wouldn't try to over-manage that part of their eating. Parents cannot act against an entire culture.

All of us who have children have noticed that, after a brief (and painful!) rebellion in adolescence, the children of Democrats usually become Democrats, those that joined religious cults generally return to the faith of their fathers, and the incorrigibles who raced motorcycles wind up driving a version of the old family station wagon.

None of us can seem to avoid sounding like our own parents as we get older, which is a shorthand way of saying that we ultimately adopt parental values. My advice, then, is to give a healthy message and model it consistently. Your children may battle you now, but in time they will see the value of your beliefs, start to live them and pass them along. Whether they have cupcakes at a birthday party or a fast food meal with friends now is not as important as what they know about their home environment and the principles that are important to you as a family.

Help on the Horizon?

One thing I have chosen not to discuss in this book is the use of weight loss medication as an aid to maintenance. Currently, we lack drugs that are forceful enough to cause large amounts of weight loss on their own. But, as you well know, weight loss is not really the problem. Most of us could summon the energy to lose the pounds if we knew there was a medication to help us maintain permanently.

Many drugs are currently under investigation. A number of studies are looking at combining available medications to allow them to work better. It may well turn out that some of these drugs offer hope for maintainers. Limited research supports the idea that maintainers taking the currently-available medicine sibutramine have an easier time keeping weight off. Some obesity doctors endorse the use of appetite suppressants such as phentermine for episodic use by maintainers.

Laws regarding prescriptions of these medicines differ from state to state. Research is not yet complete or absolutely convincing. My position is always to avoid medicines if possible. However, if you continue to struggle in maintenance, speak to your physician or bariatric specialist about whether medications are appropriate. And keep your eye out for newer forms of treatment. Many will be making appearances in the coming years.

My Wish for You

Have you ever wished you could win the lottery? Everyone enjoys that fantasy. Unfortunately, the odds are simply too staggering. In 1998, the Power Ball lottery gave away a quarter of a billion dollars. The odds for winning with one ticket were 80,000,000 to one: a pipe dream.

But here's a thought. How likely is it that you find yourself living on earth at this particular moment? The forces of the universe make lottery odds look microscopic. There are 70,000,000,000,000,000,000,000 (that's 70 sextillion!) stars in our view alone. Yet here you are.

Generation upon generation of men and women contributed the genetic material that enabled you to be. Had just one of them paired up with a different partner, the line that leads to you would have been erased.

The single biological act that created you was a competition between as many as 400 million sperm cells, each vying to become a person. Only one succeeded. That created you.

From the moment of your conception, you have been a celestial lottery winner, a true and rare miracle.

Since you've been handed a one in billions pass into this fascinating show called life, doesn't it seem a small thing to repay the universe by being a good steward of the body you've been given? To do it: eat from nature's bounty, use your incredible physical machinery and stay connected to the rhythms around you.

In this exciting and truly beautiful journey I wish you excitement, health and joy.

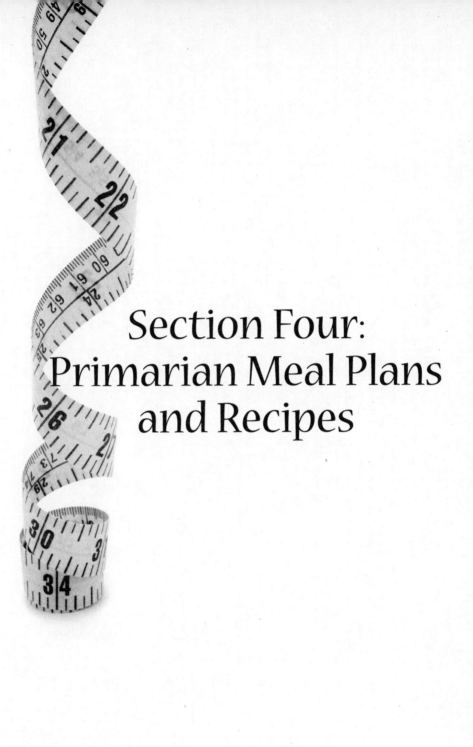

Section Four:
Primarian Meal Plans
and Recipes

Seven Primarian Days

These seven menus will give you an idea of some basic Primarian choices. Each makes use of the one major meal rule and requires limited preparation time. When choosing salad dressings, use those that contain less than twenty calories per serving. Other dressings and light mayonnaise are acceptable, if used very sparingly.

If you would like to create more flavorful and complex meals, you can find a selection of Primarian recipes designed by Chef Matthew Anderson following these seven sample days.

Day one: (Major meal at dinner)
Breakfast Mini-Meal:
Large skim-milk latte with artificial sweetener and fruit
Lunch Mini-Meal:
Large bowl of vegetable soup and a generous salad
Fast Grabs:
Unsalted nuts and fruit slices
Dinner Major Meal:
Grilled turkey burgers, large salad with many raw vegetables, broccoli, and unsweetened applesauce
Dessert:
Stewed peaches
Acceptable Treat:
Bowl of low-fat or non-fat ice cream (150 calories per serving or less)

Day two: (Major meal at lunch and eaten in a restaurant)

Breakfast Mini-Meal:

Scrambled eggs with onions, tomatoes, and peppers and a mixed fruit cup

Lunch Major Meal (restaurant):

Cup of tomato soup, grilled chicken salad, fruit salad, and a non-fat cappuccino

Fast Grabs:

Mini carrots, red and green pepper slices, and dried fruit

Dinner Mini-Meal:

Low-fat yogurt and a large baked apple

Acceptable Treat:

Low-fat, sugar-free chocolate pudding

Day three: (Major meal at dinner and in a restaurant)

Breakfast Mini-Meal:

Diet shake and coffee

Lunch Mini-Meal:

Rolled slices of turkey and sliced avocado

Fast Grabs:

Red grapes and nuts

Dinner Major Meal (restaurant):

Shrimp cocktail (easy on sauce), Caesar salad (dressing on the side—dip into it), grilled red snapper, double serving of vegetables, a glass of white wine, and coffee

Acceptable Treat:

Sugar-free jello with fruit chunks with a dollop of fat-free topping

Day four: (Major meal at dinner)

Breakfast Mini-Meal:

Light yogurt and mixed fruit

Lunch Mini-Meal:

Egg-salad, mixed salad, and a pickle

Fast Grabs:

Green beans, snow peas, and fruit slices

Dinner Major Meal:

Broiled marinated flank steak, cooked carrots, brussel sprouts, a salad of sliced beefsteak, tomato, red onion, and basil; fruits, and a glass of wine

Acceptable Treat:

Peaches stewed with nutmeg, cinnamon, and artificial sweetener with a dollop of fat-free whipped topping

Day five: (Major meal at lunch)

Breakfast Mini-Meal:

Large skim milk sugar-free mocha (add artificial sweetener if you like)

Lunch Major Meal:

Grilled salmon, a large mixed salad, asparagus, stewed tomatoes, poached pears, and coffee

Fast Grabs:

Grapes and carrots

Dinner Mini-Meal:

Deviled eggs and a salad

Acceptable Treat:

Diet ice cream cone

Day six: (Major meal is brunch)

Breakfast:

Cup of coffee

Brunch Major Meal:

Selection of vegetables and fruits, cold sliced meats, smoked salmon, and an omelet

Fast Grabs:

Unsalted nuts and dried fruit

Dinner Mini-Meal:

Bowl of soup and a salad

Acceptable Treat:

Diet ice cream sandwich

Day seven: (Major meal is dinner at a wedding)

Breakfast Mini-Meal:

Half a cantaloupe and mixed berries

Lunch Mini-Meal:

Cold sliced chicken breast and grapes

Fast Grabs:

Mini carrots and low-fat cheese sticks

Dinner Major Meal:

Glass of wine, Primarian hors d'ouvres (beef or chicken skewers, stuffed mushrooms, shrimp, crab, etc.), salad; eat the chicken or meat entree (scrape off any breading), eat the vegetable. Pass on the bread, potato, or rice and the wedding cake

Acceptable Treat:

Non-fat, low-sugar vanilla pudding over a sliced banana with a dollop of fat-free whipped topping

Primarian Recipes by Chef Matthew Anderson

Matthew Anderson currently serves as director of Pastry Arts at the International Culinary Arts and Sciences Institute in Cleveland, Ohio. He also serves as executive chef of Sapore, an international bistro. His background includes cooking stints in Washington, D.C., as executive chef at the Bluestone Café and Arlington Catering Company in Arlington, Virginia and executive sous chef at the Oval Room. His culinary interests include cooking with regional produce, and exploring local cuisine.

Chef's notes

As a chef I am often challenged by dietary restrictions. I enjoy creating dishes that will satisfy not only specific dietary needs but which are interesting and flavorful.

I hope that you will enjoy these recipes as much as I have enjoyed putting them together. They became a labor of love for me. Perhaps you too will be inspired to create wonderful Primarian foods.

Some basic assumptions: the salt is kosher and the pepper is fresh ground (either black or white will do). The herbs and the ginger should always be fresh. If possible, I suggest you use local, seasonal products as they will give the best flavor and results.

Cut vegetables uniformly and it will lower the cooking time as well as give a nicer result. Whole spices that you toast and grind yourself will yield the best flavor, but in a pinch pre-ground is fine (notice, though, that you may need more). These fresher ingredients cost a bit more, but they are going to become a part of you, and I think you're worth it.

Most importantly............enjoy!

–Matthew Anderson

Breakfast

Fruit Smoothie
1 cup non-fat yogurt
1 cup non-fat milk
2 cups ice cubes
1 cup frozen fruit
1 packet Splenda sweetener

Place all of the ingredients above into a blender and blend on high until smooth. Enjoy!

Buy a few different kinds of fruit and make your own combinations. Some tasty combinations to try:

blueberries and banana
peach and strawberry
melon and lemon zest
cherry and ¼ cup almonds
pineapple and banana

Entrées

Roasted Eggplant, No Noodle Lasagna
2 large eggplants, cut into ¼ inch slices
1 teaspoon salt
2 tablespoons olive oil

Preheat the oven to 400 degrees. Place the eggplant on a baking tray and sprinkle with half of the salt. Turn the slices over and sprinkle with the other half of the salt. Allow to drain for 30 minutes. Pour the oil over the eggplant and place eggplant in the pre-heated oven on the racks. Roast until tender, about 25-30 minutes. Remove from the oven and allow to cool.

While the eggplant is cooling make the sauce and the filling.

For the sauce:
½ cup onion, chopped
2 cloves garlic, chopped

1 teaspoon olive oil
1 teaspoon crushed red peppers
4 cups chopped tomatoes
1 cup tomato sauce
1 cup water
1 bunch fresh basil, chopped
1 teaspoon salt
½ teaspoon pepper

In a large sauce pot, cook the onions and garlic in the olive oil until tender, about 8 minutes. Add the crushed red peppers and cook for one minute. Add the chopped tomatoes, water, and the sauce. Cook for 30 minutes. Finish the sauce with basil, salt, and pepper.

Reserve the sauce. The sauce can be made up to two days in advance.

The filling:
2 cups low-fat ricotta cheese
2 eggs
1 bunch parsley, chopped
1 bunch basil, chopped
2 teaspoons pepper

Mix the above ingredients together and hold.

To assemble: Preheat the oven to 350 degrees. In a 9x13 inch baking dish, cover the bottom with a thin layer of the sauce, top with a layer of eggplant making sure the entire bottom of the pan is covered. Some slices may need to be cut to make them fit. Add a layer of the cheese filling and top with the eggplant. Continue on with layering sauce, eggplant, and filling until the pan is full, ending with a layer of sauce. Cover with foil and bake in the oven for 45 minutes. Allow the lasagna to set 15 minutes before cutting.

This lasagna can be made in steps. It can be assembled one day and baked the next.

Serves 8

Vegetable Chili

1 red onion
1 green pepper
1 yellow pepper
4 portobello mushrooms, caps only
4 cloves garlic, chopped
1 jalapeño pepper (use more if you like it hot)
1 poblano chili
1 tablespoon olive oil
2 tablespoons chili powder
1 tablespoon ground cumin
2 teaspoons smoked paprika
2 28-oz cans chopped tomatoes
1 teaspoon salt
1 teaspoon pepper
1 8-oz canned beans (ooptional)

Cut the onions, peppers, chilies, and mushrooms into ½ inch cubes. In a Dutch oven sauté the peppers, chilies, mushrooms, and garlic with the olive oil, until the vegetables are tender, about 8 minutes. Add the chili powder, cumin, and paprika. Cook for 1 minute. Add the tomatoes, salt, and pepper. Turn the heat to low and cook for 60 more minutes. Depending on the consistency you want, (and whether you have added back legumes) one 8-ounce can of beans can be added to the chili.

This chili is a great item and can be frozen. Just reheat and you have a quick meal.

Serves 6

Grilled Mushroom "Burgers" with Spicy Sour Cream

1 tablespoon ginger, chopped
1 teaspoon sesame oil
4 cloves garlic
¼ cup low-salt tamari
1 tablespoon coriander seed
1 bunch scallions
4 large portobello mushrooms, caps only

1 red onion, sliced into ¼ inch rings
1 large tomato, cut into ½ inch slices

Place the first five ingredients into a bowl and whisk to combine. Set aside. Remove the root ends of the scallions, wash well, and toss in the bowl with the marinade. Add the mushroom, onion and tomato slices. Allow the veggies to marinate for 30 minutes.

While the veggies are marinating heat the grill on medium. Drain the veggies, and reserve the marinade. Grill the veggies on medium heat until they are soft, basting with the reserved marinade. Using the mushrooms as buns, fill with vegetables and top with spicy sour cream.

Serves 4

Spicy Sour Cream
1 cup low-fat sour cream
1 teaspoon salt
½ teaspoon pepper
2 tablespoons sriricha (Asain chili garlic paste)
1 tablespoon cilantro

Mix the above ingredients together and serve. This sauce will last for up to 5 days in the refrigerator. The amount of sriricha can be adjusted based on how hot you like your food. I like it hot, so I put in 3 tablespoons.

I love the flavor of a grilled portobello mushroom. Once you have had this sandwich you won't even notice there isn't any ground beef. Sprouts, like sunflower or radish, make a great addition.

Yields 2 ¼ cups

Above Average Tuna Salad
1 8-oz can water-packed tuna
2 tablespoons sunflower seeds
1 green onion, chopped fine
¼ cup low-fat yogurt
2 tablespoons low-fat mayo
1 tablespoon curry powder
1 large apple, cut into bite size pieces

½ cup radish sprouts
1 cucumber, cut into thin slices
1 red onion, cut into thin slices
1 avocado, sliced into ¼ inch slices
1 6-oz bag lettuce, cleaned
Fresh ground pepper

Mix the first six ingredients together. Divide the salad greens among 4 plates and top with the remaining ingredients. Finish with a big twist of black pepper.

This is a different take on the usual tuna salad. It has nice crunch and the apple lends a little sweetness.

Serves 4

South of the Border Salmon

1 tablespoon cumin
2 tablespoons chili powder
½ tablespoon black pepper
¼ teaspoon salt
¼ teaspoon cinnamon
¼ teaspoon cloves
1 teaspoon cayenne
2 teaspoons coriander

Mix the ingredients above together and place in an airtight container. Store in a dark place. Pre-ground spices are fine to use here, but for the best flavor purchase whole spices, toast them and grind them yourself. It's a bit more work, but you really can't compare for flavor.

4 4-oz pieces salmon
2 tablespoons of the above seasoning mix
½ cup low-fat yogurt
1 lime, zested and juiced
1 teaspoon olive oil
1 clove garlic, minced
2 bunches cilantro, picked and washed, stems removed
2 bunches watercress, or any peppery green
2 tablespoons pepitas (toasted pumpkin seeds)

½ teaspoon salt
¼ teaspoon pepper

Preheat the grill on high heat. Blend the seasoning mix with the yogurt and lime juice and spread all over the fish. Allow to marinate for 15 minutes. Cook the fish on the grill until desired doneness. 4-5 minutes per side. While the salmon is cooking, heat a large sauté pan over medium. Add the oil and cook the garlic until it is just brown, add the cilantro and stir to coat with the oil, add the watercress, salt and pepper, and cook until the greens are just wilted. Add the pepitas and lime zest. Serve at once with the grilled fish.

This is a great summer dish. Look for pepitas in any South American or specialty grocery store. Sunflower seeds make a fine alternative. The greens really need to be cooked just a little. Crunchy is good. I usually cook this more like a stir-fry. Quick high heat and just wilted.

Serves 4

White Wine Steamed Trout

8 fillets of trout, boneless
½ cup white wine
Juice of one lemon
1 teaspoon butter
1 carrot, cut into thin strips
½ cup onion, cut into thin strips
¼ teaspoon capers
1 tablespoon kalamata olives
2 tomatoes, cut into quarters
1 bunch asparagus, cleaned, tough ends removed
4 sprigs thyme
½ teaspoon black pepper

Preheat the oven to 350 degrees. Mix the carrot, onion, capers, and olives together. With the teaspoon of butter, grease the sides and bottom of a 9x13 inch pan. Spread the carrots and onions evenly on the bottom, then add the asparagus in a single layer. Place the trout fillets in the pan, forming an "X" with two fillets. There should be 4 "Xs" spaced evenly in the pan. Add the tomato quarters, white wine, and lemon juice. Place a thyme sprig on the top of each "X." Cover the pan with foil and place in the preheated oven. Bake until the fish is cooked and the vegetables are tender, about 20 minutes. Remove the thyme sprigs and enjoy.

This is a great summertime dish. It can be made with salmon fillets just as easily.

Serves 4

Side Dishes

Stuffed Tomatoes

6 large tomatoes
¼ teaspoon salt

Cut the tops of the tomatoes off and scoop out the seeds. Season the inside and turn upside down on a wire rack and allow to drain for 2 minutes. While they are draining make the filling.

The filling:

1 teaspoon olive oil
½ cup onion, chopped fine
4 cups spinach, washed and chopped
1 cup low-fat ricotta cheese
1 egg
2 tablespoons walnuts, chopped
2 tablespoons parsley, chopped

In a large sauté pan over medium heat, cook the onions and spinach with the olive oil until the onions are soft, about 10 minutes. Cool and mix with the remaining ingredients. Divide evenly between the tomatoes and stuff with the filling. At this point the tomatoes can be refrigerated overnight.

When you're ready to cook, preheat the oven to 350 degrees. Place the tomatoes in a baking dish and bake for 25-30 minutes or until the tomatoes are soft and the filling is hot.

Feta cheese is a great addition to this dish. Pine nuts can be used instead of walnuts.

Serves 6

Curried Cauliflower

¼ cup onion, chopped
2 cloves garlic, chopped
2 teaspoons ginger, chopped
1 tablespoon olive oil
1 head cauliflower, cut into small pieces
1 tablespoon curry powder (you can use more if you really
    like curry)
¼ cup golden raisins
¼ cup pine nuts
1 cup water
2 cups spinach, cut into ribbons

In a medium sauce pot, over medium heat, sauté the onion, garlic, and ginger in the olive oil. Cook until the onions are soft, about 8 minutes. Add the cauliflower and cook for 5 more minutes. Add the curry and cook for 1 more minute. Add the raisins, pine nuts, and water. Cover and turn the heat to low and cook until the cauliflower is tender, about 10 more minutes, depending on the size. Once the cauliflower is tender, add the spinach and allow to wilt.

This dish can be prepaired in advance. Prepare up through the cooking of the cauliflower. When ready to eat, reheat and toss in spinach as described above.

Serves 4

Summer Vegetable Ragout

1 small zucchini
1 small summer squash
1 eggplant
1 head fennel
½ cup onion, chopped
2 tablespoons garlic, chopped
2 teaspoons olive oil
1 cup canned tomatoes, chopped
Water as needed
1 teaspoon salt
¼ teaspoon pepper
Zest of one lemon

¼ cup basil, cut into thin ribbons

The success of this dish and its quick cooking time rely on the cutting of the vegetables. They all need to be cut to about the same size, ½ inch cubes. For the eggplant: cut into pieces smaller than the rest. Fresh tomatoes are great when they are in season, but canned are just fine.

In a large sauté pan, cook the onion and garlic in the olive oil until tender, about 8 minutes. Add the zucchini, summer squash, eggplant, and fennel. Cook for 10 minutes on medium heat. Add the tomatoes. Add water if needed to bring the level of the liquid above the vegetables in the pan. Add the salt and pepper. Turn the heat to low and cook until the vegetables are tender and the sauce is thick, about 15 minutes. Add the zest and basil.

This ragout can be prepared in advance and then reheated. Add the lemon zest and basil when reheating. This ragout is actually better after a day in the refrigerator. It can also be served at room temperature.

Serves 4

Roasted Eggplant with Sesame

2 large eggplants, peeled and cut into ½-inch match sticks
1 teaspoon salt
½ onion, sliced into ½ inch rings
1 tablespoon garlic, chopped
1 tablespoon ginger, chopped
1 tablespoon sesame oil
1 bunch scallions, whites and green parts sliced thin
Juice of two limes
2 teaspoons sesame seeds (white or black)

Preheat the oven to 350 degrees. Once the eggplants are cut, toss with the salt and allow to drain in a colander for 30 minutes. Squeeze out the excess moisture and toss in a bowl with the onions, garlic, ginger, and sesame oil. Place on a baking tray and cook in the oven until the eggplant is tender, about 25-30 minutes. Turn the eggplant once or twice with a spatula to promote even browning. Once the eggplant is tender, remove from the oven and toss with the sesame seeds, scallions, and lime juice.

This dish is great hot from the oven, but is great at room temperature also.

Serves 4

Mashed turnips and parsnips

½ pound parsnips, peeled and cut into 1 inch pieces
½ pound turnips, peeled and cut into 1 inch cubes
2 cups milk
1 stick cinnamon
1 piece star anise
2 tablespoons greek yogurt
2 teaspoons salt
1 teaspoon pepper

Place the turnips and parsnips in a pot large enough to hold them. Add one cup of the milk, the star anise, cinnamon stick, and 1 teaspoon of salt. Cover with water, bring to a boil, and cook until the vegetables are tender. Drain and return to the heat. Heat the vegetables for a few minutes to dry out, stirring the whole time. Push the vegetables through a potato ricer to make a smooth puree. Add the rest of the milk, salt, greek yogurt, and the pepper. Return to the heat and warm to serve.

Serves 4

Roasted Lemon Asparagus

1 bunch asparagus, trimmed
¼ cup water
1 lemon, zested and juiced
1 egg, hard boiled and grated
¼ cup parsley, chopped
¼ cup low-fat parmesan cheese, grated
2 tablespoons olive oil
½ teaspoon olive oil
¼ teaspoon black pepper

Preheat the oven to 350 degrees. Place the asparagus in a baking dish, add the water and cover with foil. Bake in the oven until the asparagus is tender, about 5-8 minutes. While the asparagus is cooking, mix the remaining ingredients together. Uncover the asparagus and turn the oven up to 400 degrees. Cover the asparagus with the crumb topping and bake in the oven until golden brown. Serve at once.

Serves 4

Salads

Roasted Carrot Salad with Coriander Vinaigrette

For the salad:

    4 cups carrots, peeled and cut into bite size pieces

    1 small onion, sliced thin

    ½ teaspoon ground coriander seed

    ½ teaspoon salt

    ¼ teaspoon ground pepper

Preheat the oven to 400 degrees. In a large bowl, toss the carrots, onion, olive oil, coriander, salt, and pepper. Place on a baking tray and roast in the oven until the carrots are tender. About 30 minutes. Remove from the oven and allow to cool.

While the carrots are roasting, make the vinaigrette.

For the vinaigrette:

    ½ cup low-fat yogurt

    2 tablespoons olive oil

    ¼ cup fresh cilantro leaves, chopped

    ¼ cup parsley leaves, chopped

    1 ½ tablespoons fresh lemon juice

    ½ teaspoon salt

    ¼ teaspoon ground black pepper

    ⅛ teaspoon cayenne pepper

Mix the ingredients for the vinaigrette in a bowl. Toss with the cooled carrots and allow the flavors to develop for 30 minutes.

This salad can be made up to 2 days before it is needed.

It is a tasty alternative to potato salad.

Warm Spinach Salad with Spiced Pecans and Sherry Vinaigrette

For the vinaigrette:

    1 tablespoon onion, chopped

    1 clove garlic, chopped

    ¼ cup sherry vinegar

¾ cup olive oil

1 tablespoon Dijon mustard

1 teaspoon Splenda sweetener

½ teaspoon salt

¼ teaspoon pepper

Whisk the ingredients above together and store covered in the refrigerator until ready to use. This vinaigrette will last up to one week in your refrigerator.

Yields 1 ½ cups

For the pecans:

1 cup pecans

1 teaspoon salt

½ tablespoon paprika

½ tablespoon chili powder

½ teaspoon ground cumin

½ teaspoon cayenne

1 teaspoon Splenda

1 tablespoon water

Preheat the oven to 350 degrees. Toss the ingredients for the pecans together and spread onto a cookie sheet. Bake in the oven until the nuts are golden brown, about 20 minutes. Store the nuts in an airtight container until ready to use. The nuts will store on the shelf for up to 2 weeks.

Yields 1 cup

For the salad:

1 pound baby spinach, cleaned

¼ cup sherry vinaigrette

¼ cup spiced pecans

In a 10 inch sauté pan over low heat warm the vinaigrette until it just begins to bubble. Add the spinach and toss to coat well, allow the spinach to just wilt. Add the pecans and serve at once. Grilled chicken or lean fish can be added on top of the salad for a quick lunch or a light dinner.

Serves 4

Marinated Fennel and Leek Salad with Smoked Salmon

8 oz smoked salmon

2 bulbs fennel, tops removed and shaved thin
1 leek, white part only sliced into thin ribbons
1 carrot peeled, cut into match-sticks

Place the vegetables into a bowl.

For the marinade:
1 teaspoon Splenda
1 teaspoon thyme, chopped
½ teaspoon pepper
Juice of one lemon
½ cup white vinegar

In a small saucepan, bring the ingredients for the marinade to a boil. Once boiling, pour it over the vegetables and cover with plastic wrap. Allow the salad to cool.

Once the salad is cool it can be stored covered in the refrigerator for 2 days.

To serve the salad:
For each person you will need 2 ounces smoked salmon. Arrange some of the vegetables on a plate and lay the smoked salmon attractively on the top. Serve at once.

This salad is a wonderful first course or a great light salad on a warm day, when using the stove seems like too much work.

A note on leeks: Leeks grow in very sandy soil. As a result, once they are cut they need to be washed well. I often soak them in two or three changes of water. Once there is no more grit at the bottom of the sink, they are clean.

A note on fennel: Fennel has a wonderful, anise flavor. It's very refreshing.

Serves 4

Artichoke and Red Onion with Whole Grain Mustard

2 12-oz cans of artichoke hearts

1 red onion, cut into thin slices

1 rib of celery, chopped

1 red pepper, sliced into thin strips

1 tablespoon sage, chopped

Juice of one lemon

2 tablespoons whole grain mustard

¼ cup olive oil

½ teaspoon ground pepper

Drain the artichokes and rinse under cold water. Pat dry and cut into quarters. Toss with the remaining ingredients and let the flavors develop for at least 30 minutes.

If you are using fresh artichokes, you will need 10.

Cover the fresh artichokes with cold water. Add two lemons cut up and bring the artichokes to a simmer over medium heat. Cook the artichokes until tender, about 45 minutes. Allow to cool in the water. Then peel the leaves back until you reach the heart. Remove the soft choke with a spoon and rinse well. Cut the hearts into quarters and continue on with the recipe.

This salad is a great accompaniment to grilled beef or lamb.

Serves 6

Zucchini and Cucumber Salad

2 large cucumbers, peeled, seeded, and cut into half-moons

1 zucchini, cut into half-moons

½ teaspoon salt

¼ cup white vinegar

4 large tomatoes, seeded and cut into bite size pieces

½ cup red onion, sliced thinly

2 teaspoons olive oil

¼ teaspoon ground pepper

2 tablespoons mint, chopped

2 tablespoons parsley, chopped

Toss the cucumber and the zucchini with the salt and vinegar. Marinate 15 minutes. Drain and toss with the tomatoes and onions. Add the olive oil, pepper, mint, and parsley. Serve at once.

This makes a tasty accompaniment to grilled shrimp, scallops, or beef.
Serves 4 as a side dish

Greek Salad

1 cucumber, peeled, seeded, and cut into cubes
1 large tomato, seeded and cut into bite size pieces
1 red onion, cut into rings
¼ cup low-fat feta cheese
¼ cup kalamata olives
1 head romaine lettuce, washed and cut into ribbons

Toss the above ingredients together and arrange attractively on a platter. Serve with Greek Vinaigrette.

Greek Vinaigrette:
¼ cup red wine vinegar
Juice of two lemons
2 teaspoons dried oregano
2 cloves garlic, minced
1 cup olive oil
3 tablespoons fresh oregano

Combine the above ingredients and allow the flavors to develop for 30 minutes if possible.
Yields 1½ cups

For a heartier lunch or a light dinner, grilled fish or chicken can be added to this. I often add a can of tuna to this salad for a change of pace.
Serves 4 as a light lunch

Marinades, Relishes

Orange and Tomato Relish

1 cup fresh tomatoes, seeded and chopped

1 6-oz can mandarin oranges, drained
¼ cup red onion, minced
1 clove garlic, minced
1 tablespoon fresh orange juice
1 tablespoon mint, chopped
½ teaspoon salt
¼ teaspoon pepper
1 tablespoon olive oil

Mix the above ingredients together, cover, and chill for at least 30 minutes before using.

Fresh oranges can be used for this relish. Peel and remove flesh from the fruit. Ruby red grapefruit make a wonderful addition to this relish also.

This relish can be made and stored for up to 4 days in the refrigerator. It is a great addition to grilled fish or chicken.

Yields 1 ¾ cups

Roasted Red Pepper Chutney

4 red peppers, roasted, peeled, and sliced into thin strips
4 cloves garlic, minced
¼ cup red onion, minced
1 teaspoon olive oil
1 tablespoon curry powder
1 cup apple cider
¼ cup dried cherries
½ cup rice wine vinegar
Juice of 1 orange
Juice of 1 lemon
2 tablespoons cilantro, chopped

In a medium saucepan, sauté the first four ingredients until the onions are tender.

Add the curry powder and cook for 1 minute. Add the apple cider, then turn the heat to high and cook until the cider is reduced by ¾, stirring constantly. Add the dried cherries, rice wine vinegar, orange, and lemon juice and cook for 2 more minutes. Turn off the heat and add the cilantro.

This chutney will keep refrigerated for up to one week. The level of curry powder can be adjusted and if you like it spicy, add one chopped jalapeño to the onion and sauté.

This makes a great accompaniment to grilled lamb or beef.

Yields about 3 cups

Indian Spiced Yogurt

2 tablespoons olive oil
2 large onions, sliced thin
2 teaspoons garlic, minced
1 teaspoon ginger, minced
1 teaspoon mustard powder
1 teaspoon fennel powder
1 teaspoon cumin powder
1 teaspoon red chile powder
1 teaspoon turmeric powder
1 teaspoon salt
1 cup low-fat yogurt
Juice of 1 lime or lemon
Salt to taste

In a small sauté pan over medium heat, cook the onion, garlic, and ginger with the olive oil until the onions are soft. Add the mustard, fennel, cumin, chile, and turmeric. Cook for 2 more minutes to release the flavors in the spices. Remove from the heat and allow to cool completely before adding the yogurt and the lime juice. Cover and store in the refrigerator until needed.

This makes a great dip for vegetables. It can also be used as a marinade for lamb chops, pork, or beef. If you are using it as a marinade, do not allow it to stay on the meat for more than 4 hours. Do not remove marinade from the meat, just cook it in the oven for a wonderful flavor.

Yields about 1 ½ cups

Walnut Pesto

1 cup walnuts, toasted

¼ cup olive oil
1 cup fresh basil leaves
1 cup fresh parsley leaves
2 cloves garlic
½ teaspoon salt
¼ teaspoon pepper
2 tablespoons parmesan cheese

In the bowl of a food processor, add the olive oil, garlic, and walnuts. Pulse until the walnuts and garlic are chopped. Add the herbs and run the machine until the herbs are chopped. Add the cheese and the salt and pepper. Store covered in the refrigerator until needed.

The amount of time that you let the food processor run is up to you. If you want a chunky pesto, don't run the machine very long. For a smoother consistency, run the machine longer.

This makes a great accompaniment to grilled fish, or a nice dip for roasted vegetables. Sometimes I will toss some in the Roasted Eggplant Lasagna, or on top of my Mushroom Burger. Enjoy.

Yields about 2 cups

Soups

Tomato Gazpacho
1 cup fresh tomatoes, chopped
½ cup zucchini, chopped
½ cup onion, chopped
1 clove garlic, chopped
½ cup tomato vegetable juice
2 tablespoons cider vinegar
1 teaspoon jalapeño, chopped
1 cup cucumber, peeled chopped, and seeds removed
¼ teaspoon salt
¼ teaspoon fresh ground pepper

In the jar of a blender, combine the above ingredients and puree until smooth. Allow to chill for 30 minutes and serve.

Yields 4 cups

Puree of Cauliflower Soup

1 head cauliflower, with the core removed and cut into small
  pieces
½ cup onion, chopped
1 clove of garlic, chopped
2 teaspoons ginger, peeled and chopped
1 bay leaf
½ teaspoon thyme, chopped
1 teaspoon olive oil
6 cups vegetable stock
½ teaspoon salt
¼ teaspoon pepper
1 tablespoon fresh chives, chopped

In a large stockpot, heat the olive oil over low heat. Add the onions, garlic, and ginger and cook until the onions are soft, stirring often, about 8 minutes. Add the cauliflower and cook for an additional 10 minutes, while continuing to stir. Add the bay leaf, thyme, vegetable stock, salt, and pepper. Cover the pot with a tight fitting lid and turn the heat up to medium. Cook until the cauliflower is soft, about 15 minutes.

Once the vegetables are soft, turn the heat off and remove the bay leaf. Puree the soup in a blender in small batches. Reheat the soup and serve with the chives for garnish.

This soup makes a nice sized batch for a family, with some leftover to freeze.

Yields 8 cups

Tomato Basil Soup

4 cups fresh tomatoes, chopped with seeds removed
1 cup onion, chopped
2-4 cloves garlic
1 carrot, chopped
¼ cup fresh basil leaves, chopped
2 teaspoons olive oil
½ teaspoon salt
¼ teaspoon pepper
2 tablespoons fresh basil leaves cut into thin ribbons

In a large stockpot over medium heat, sauté the onion, garlic, and carrots in the olive oil until the vegetables are soft, about 8 minutes. Add the tomatoes, basil, salt, and pepper and continue to cook for 15 more minutes, or until the vegetables are very soft. Remove from the heat and in small batches puree the soup to the desired consistency. Return to the heat and bring to a boil, garnish with the 2 tablespoons of basil ribbons and serve at once.

Yields 6 cups

Curried Winter Vegetable Soup

1 cup carrots, chopped
½ cup celery, chopped
½ cup onion, chopped
1 cup parsnip, chopped
1 cup red beets, chopped
1 cup cabbage, shredded
1 cup turnip, chopped
1 clove garlic, minced
1 teaspoon ginger, minced
1 tablespoon olive oil
1 tablespoon good quality curry powder
8 cups vegetable stock or water
2 teaspoons salt
1 teaspoon ground pepper
1 cup fresh spinach cut into thin ribbons

In a large stockpot over medium heat, cook the first nine ingredients in the olive oil until the onions are soft, stirring often. About 10 minutes. Add the curry powder and cook for 2 more minutes. Add the stock and bring to a simmer. Add the salt and pepper and cook until the vegetables are tender. About 15 minutes. Add the spinach and serve at once.

Notes: The quick cooking time of this soup relies on the vegetables being all about the same size. Also if you don't like one of the vegetables I have mentioned here, feel free to omit it. Tomatoes make a nice addition to this soup and the curry can be omitted as well if curry isn't your thing.

Serves 6

Spicy Chicken Soup

½ cup onion, chopped
½ cup celery, chopped
½ cup carrot, chopped
1-2 jalapeños, seeds removed and chopped
1 teaspoon ginger, chopped
1 clove garlic, chopped
1 teaspoon sesame oil
4 cups chicken stock
1 inch piece fresh lemon grass
1 cup cooked chicken breast, diced
¼ teaspoon salt
¼ teaspoon pepper
½ cup snow peas
2 tablespoons fresh cilantro leaves

In a large stockpot over medium heat, cook the first six ingredients in the sesame oil until the onions are soft, about 5-8 minutes. Add the stock and bring to a simmer, then add the lemongrass and the chicken breast. Turn the heat to low and cook until the vegetables are tender. Add the salt and pepper. Garnish with the snow peas and cilantro and serve at once.

Notes: This soup can be as spicy as you like by adjusting the amount of jalapeño you add. A great substitution for the lemongrass is lemon zest.

Serves 4

Hot and Sour Soup

1 tablespoon ginger, finely chopped
1 tablespoon garlic, finely chopped
¼ cup onion, sliced thin
2 teaspoons fresh jalapeño, sliced thin
2 teaspoons olive oil
½ inch piece lemongrass
2 kaffir lime leaves
1 pound shrimp, peeled and deveined (any size will do)
   (or 1 cup cooked chicken breast cut into small cubes)
4 cups chicken or shrimp stock
2 tablespoons rice wine vinegar
1 teaspoon Splenda sweetener

¼ cup fish sauce
½ cup fresh mushrooms sliced
   (straw or shiitake add a nice flavor, but almost any mushroom will do)

In a large stockpot over a medium flame, heat the olive oil. Add the garlic, ginger, jalapeño, and onion. Sautee until the ginger becomes fragrant. Add the lemongrass and kaffir lime leaves cooking 2 more minutes. Add the shrimp, or the chicken, and cook just until the shrimp are pink, about 3 minutes, or the chicken is fully cooked. Add the stock and bring to a simmer. Add the Splenda, vinegar, fish sauce, and mushrooms, allowing the mixture to simmer for 5 more minutes. Remove the lemongrass and the lime leaves and serve at once.

This soup is quick and very flavorful. It can easily be made vegetarian, by omitting the shrimp and/or chicken and by using vegetable stock.

If lemongrass is not available, the zest and juice of 2 lemons can be used. If kaffir leaves are not available, the juice and zest of 1 lime can be used. Lemongrass and kaffir leaves are avilable in Asian markets and many gourmet grocery stores.

Yields 8 cups

Desserts

Toasted Nut Soufflé
¾ cup toasted nuts
½ cup Splenda
1 tablespoon fresh lemon juice
4 egg whites
3 tablespoons nut flour
1 teaspoon butter

Preheat the oven to 375 degrees. Butter and coat a 2 cup soufflé pan with 1 tablespoon of the nut flour, set aside.

Coarsely chop the nuts and mix with the Splenda. Toss with the lemon juice and remaining nut flour. Place the mixture into a food processor and blend until smooth. Whip the egg whites until stiff and fold in the nut mixture, pour the mix into the prepared soufflé pan.

Place the soufflé pan in a shallow pan and fill the shallow pan half full with warm water. Place in the preheated oven and bake for 20-25 minutes or until the soufflé is puffed and brown on top. Serve at once.

Any type of nuts will work for this soufflé. Nut flours can be purchased at most specialty food stores.

This soufflé needs to be served at once or it will fall and won't look as nice.

Serves 2-3

Stuffed Baked Apple
4 large cooking apples
¼ cup chestnut flour
1 teaspoon butter
½ cup English walnuts, chopped
½ teaspoon almond extract
zest of 1 lemon
½ cup applesauce
1 egg yolk
1 teaspoon ground cinnamon
1 cinnamon stick
½ teaspoon ground nutmeg
¼ teaspoon ground ginger
1 piece star anise
1 cup apple cider

Preheat the oven to 375 degrees. Use an apple corer to remove the core and some of the apple flesh. Do not peel the apples.

Mix the next seven ingredients together. Add the ground cinnamon, nutmeg, and ginger to the filling. Divide the mixture into four equal portions and stuff each apple.

Place the apples in a 9x9 inch pan. Add the cinnamon sticks, star anise, and apple cider. Cover the pan with foil and bake until the apples are tender, about 45 minutes. Remove the apples from the pan and pour the cooking liquid into a small pot. Cook over medium heat until the sauce is reduced by one half. Serve with the apples.

Choose apples that are hard (what is called a "cooking apple"). I like Fuji, Crispin, or Mitsu.

Chestnut flour can be found at some Italian specialty markets, or at grocery stores around Christmas time. Any nut flour can be substituted. The chestnut flour adds a nice sweetness to the apple, however.

Serves 4

Caramelized Peaches

4 large peaches
1 teaspoon butter
¼ teaspoon ground cinnamon
1 teaspoon fresh ginger, chopped
1 cup peach nectar

Choose firm peaches. Slice the fruit in half, remove the pits, and cut into ¼ inch slices.

In a medium sauté pan over high heat, cook the peaches with the butter until they are nice and brown and just beginning to soften. Add the ginger and cook for 1 minute. Add the cinnamon and peach nectar. Turn the heat to low and cook until the peaches are very soft. Remove the peaches from the pan, turn the heat up to high and reduce the liquid until it becomes thick. Add the peaches back to the sauté pan and stir to coat the fruit.

Almost any fruit can be used if peaches are not available.

Peach nectar can be found at many health food stores; apple cider is a fine alternative.

Serves 4

Grilled Pineapple with Cardamom Yogurt

1 large pineapple
2 cups fresh pineapple juice
1 teaspoon cayenne pepper
½ teaspoon salt
2 tablespoons olive oil

Preheat the grill on high, also preheat the oven to 350 degrees.

Cut the top and the bottom off the pineapple, remove the peel, lay the pineapple down on its long side, and cut slices ½ inch thick. Mix the cayenne, salt, and olive oil together and brush both sides of the pineapple slices. Place on the grill and allow the fruit to cook for 4-5 minutes on each side. The pineapple will not be cooked through, but it will have a wonderful flavor from the grill. Place the grilled pineapple slices in an ovenproof baking dish, add the pineapple juice and cover with foil. Place in the preheated oven and bake until the pineapple is fork tender, about 25 minutes. Remove the pineapple from the pan and pour the liquid into a small sauté pan. Cook the liquid over medium heat until the sauce thickens, about 10 minutes, stirring constantly. Reserve 2 tablespoons of the sauce for the cardamom yogurt, serve the rest with the pineapple.

Cardamom Yogurt:
>   2 cups low-fat yogurt
>   1 teaspoon ground cardamom
>   2 tablespoons pineapple sauce reserved from the cooked pineapple above

Stir these ingredients together and serve with the grilled pineapple.
Serves 6

Melon Sherbet

2 small cantaloupes
¼ cup Splenda
1 ½ cups water
2 tablespoons lemon juice
¼ cup white wine
2 egg whites (use pasteurized egg whites, available in the frozen food section of most super markets)

Halve the melons, remove the seeds, and scoop out the flesh. Save the rinds and place them in the freezer to use for serving. Puree the flesh in a blender and measure out 2 cups of puree. Mix together the melon puree, water, Splenda, lemon juice, and white wine. Place in a metal 9x13 inch pan and put it in the freezer. Stir with a wire whisk every hour or so to help create a smooth texture. Once it is about half frozen, whip the egg whites to peaks and fold into the melon mixture. Return the mixture to the freezer and freeze until the desired consistency is reached. Using a spoon to scrape the mixture, fill the reserved melon shells and serve at once.

This process can take about 4 hours. It is recommended that you start well in advance of the time the sherbet is needed.

Any ripe melon will give you the desired flavor.
Serves 4

Recommended Reading

Eat, Drink and Be Healthy, Walter Willett, M.D., Free Press, NY, 2001

Good Calories, Bad Calories, Gary Taubes, Alfred A. Knopf, NY, 2007

In Defense of Food: An Eater's Manifesto, Michael Pollan, Penguin Press, NY, 2008

Mindless Eating, Brian Wansink, Ph.D., Bantam Books, NY, 2006 NY, 2002

The Omnivore's Dilemma, Michael Pollan, Penguin Books, NY, 2006

The Paleo Diet, Loren Cordain, Ph.D, John Wiley & Sons, Hoboken,

The Paleolithic Prescription, S. Boyd Eaton, Marjorie Shostak, Melvin Konner, Harper and Row, NY, 1988

What to Eat, Marion Nestle, North Point Press, NY, 2006

Websites

americangrassfed.org (Search for grassfed beef producers in your area.)

americangrassfedbeef.com (Under "articles—Grass-fed beef," see the section entitled, "Does your grass fed beef pass the test?" for a list of questions to ask when purchasing.)

beyondveg.com (Search for Paleolithic Diet to find a wealth of references and material on ancient eating.)

cdc.gov/nccdphp/dnpa/bmi (Calculate your BMI (body mass index) on the CDC website.)

freewebs.com/lynnsjourney , (Lynn Bering's weight loss blog.)

hsph.harvard.edu/nutritionsource (Harvard School of Public Health nutrition site. Contains excellent, up-to-date, well-documented information on nutrition research.)

nwcr.ws (Site of the National Weight Control Registry.)

paleodiet.com (Much more info on the same.)

refusetoregain.typepad.com (A companion site for this book which provides ongoing education, support, and community to maintainers.)

staffanlindeberg.com (A physician and researcher's site on Paleolithic eating.)

thepaleodiet.com (Dr. Loren Cordain's website and an excellent resource.)

weightmanagementpartners.com (Dr. Berkeley's practice website. Contains a video in which she explains metabolic syndrome.)

weightwatchers.com (Registered members have access to a slew of message boards that share inspiration, support, and advice.)

Other Resources

- Ice blankets used by Carla in her readi-pak: Made by Cryopak. Available at Kmart or through Amazon.com.
- OPTIFAST®: Meal replacements used for dieting and maintenance. Available only through registered OPTIFAST® programs (Nestlé HealthCare Nutrition, Inc). To find the one nearest you, log on to OPTIFAST.com. Programs may be willing to take you on as a maintainer. Once registered, you will be able to use OPTIFAST® in your program as a meal replacement once or twice a day.
- Walden Farms no calorie dressing packs. Can be ordered on their website at waldenfarms.com.

Resources

Refuse to Regain! Wallet Card

Make a photocopy of this page then trim out the card for your wallet.

The 12 Tough Rules

1. Be Tough, Not Moderate
2. Commit Yourself to a Three-Month Opt Out Period
3. Weigh Yourself Every Day
4. Reverse Small Regains Immediately
5. Eat Primarian 90 Percent of the Time
6. Eat One Major Meal per Day
7. Perform a Daily Scan and Plan
8. Stop Eating at 8 P.M.
9. Eat From a Limited Menu
10. Have One Acceptable Treat per Day
11. Have a Love Affair with Exercise
12. Maintain with Support and Support Others

←Fold
here

Rules of Primarian Eating

Eat the following while staying below Scream Weight:
- Lean meats, fish, skinless poultry, seafood
- Vegetables and non-starchy legumes
- Fruits
- Non-caloric drinks

Eat the following sparingly:
- Eggs (up to 6 per week)
- Unsalted nuts and seeds
- Low-fat or non-fat dairy products
- Olive, flax, canola oils

Avoid the following 90 percent of the time:
- Starches (grains, cereals, bread, corn, potatoes, pasta, rice, flour, etc.)
- Sugar and other sweetners
- Sweets (cake, candy, cookies, etc.)
- Packaged foods with long, complicated ingredient lists
- Salt (use modest amounts in cooking only)

References

"Accepted/Applied Charts of Medical School Applicants." Cornell Career Services. Cornell University. http://www.career.cornell.edu/HealthCareers/acceptedApplied.html.

Annual Report, McDonald's 2006. 23 Sept. 2007 http://www.McDonald's.com.

Amatruda, JM, Statt, MC, and Welle, SL. "Total and Resting Energy Expenditure In Obese Women Reduced to Ideal Body Weight." *Journal of Clinical Investigation*, 1993;92: 1236-1242.

Aronne, Louis, et al. *A Practical Guide to Drug-Induced Weight Gain*. New York: McGraw-Hill, 2002.

Bernardo, Rosemary. "Long Distance Love Affair." *Star Bulletin*. 12 Dec. 2005.

Blanchet, Kevin. "Public Health News." *Obesity Management*, 2005; 1(4): 176-180.

Bouchard, Claude, et al. "The Response to Long-Term Overfeeding in Identical Twins." *New England Journal of Medicine*, 1990 May; 322 (21):1477-1482.

Boyle, JP, et al. "Projection of Diabetes Burden Through 2050: Impact of Changing Demography and Disease Prevalence in the US." *Diabetes Care*, 2001; 24 (11): 1936-1940.

Brownell, Kelly. *Food Fight*. New York: McGraw-Hill, 2004.

Burger King Facts. 22 Jan. 2008 http://www.Burger King.com.

Burroughs, V, and Nonas, C. "Managing Patient Risks During Weight Loss." *Obesity Management*, 2006 Apr: 63-66.

"Caloric Values of Alcoholic Beverages." University of Rochester Health Promotion Office. http://www.rochester.edu/uhs/healthtopics/Alcohol/caloricvalues.html.

"Calcium and Milk." *Nutrition Source*, Harvard School of Public Health. http://www.hsph.harvard.edu/nutritionsource/what-should-you-eat/calcium-and-milk/index.html.

Campbell, T. Colin, PhD, and Campbell, Thomas M. *The China Study*. Dallas: Benbella Books, 2006.

Cancer and Obesity Facts, NAASO. The Obesity Society. 26 Mar. 2007 http://www.naaso.org//_obesity.asp.

Cancer Prevalence Statistics. 10 Aug. 2007, http://www.seer.cancer.gov//_2004/_single/_02_table.16.pdf.

CDC National Center for Health Statistics. 18 Jan. 2008 http://www.cdc.gov/nchs/fastats/Default.htm.

"CDC National Diabetes Fact Sheet." CDC. http://www.diabetes.org/uedocuments/NationalDiabetesFactSheetRev.pdf.

Cherkas, Lynn F. PhD, et al. "The Association Between Physical Activity in Leisure Time and Leukocyte Telomere Length." *Archives of Internal Medicine*, 2008;168(2): 154-158.

Christakis, N., and Fowler, J. "The Spread of Obesity In a Large Social Network Over 32 Years." *New England Journal of Medicine*, 2007 Jul 26; 357(4): 370-379.

Church, T., Earnest, C., et al. "Effects of Different Doses of Physical Activity on Cardiorespiratory Fitness Among Sedentary Overweight and Obese Postmenopausal Women With Elevated Blood Pressure." *Journal of the American Medical Association*, 2007; 297: 2081-2091.

Colantuoni, et al. "Evidence That Intermittent, Excessive Sugar Intake Causes Endogenous Opioid Dependence." *Obesity Research*, 2002; 10:478-488.

Cordain, L. "The Nutritional Characteristics of a Contemporary Diet Based Upon Paleolithic Food Groups." *Journal of the American Neutraceutical Association,_2002*; 5: 15-24.

Cordain, Loren, et al. "Origins and Evolution of the Western Diet: Health Implications for the 21st Century." *American Journal of Clinical Nutrition*, Feb 2005; 81 (2): 341-354.

Cordain, Loren, PhD. *The Paleo Diet*. New York: John Wiley and Sons, 2002.

Cordain. Loren, PhD, Friel, J. *The Paleo Diet for Athletes*. Rodale, 2005.

Deen, Darwin, MD, MS. "Metabolic Syndrome: Time for Action." *American Family Physician*, 2004 Jun 15; 69 (12):2875-82.

DeLorenzo, A, et al. "Normal-Weight Obese Syndrome: Early Inflammation?" *American Journal of Clinical Nutrition*, 2007;85: 40-45.

Diamond, Jared. "The Worst Mistake in the History of the Human Race." *Discover*. May 1987: 64-66.

References

Dillon, Sam. "Troubles Grow for a University Built on Profits." *The New York Times*. 11 Feb. 2007.

Drezner, Daniel. "The Graduate School Crisis." *The Chicago Tribune*. 20 Apr. 2007 http://www.danieldrezner.com/archives/001064.html

Early, J., C. Apovian, et al. "Sibutramine Plus Meal Replacement Therapy For Body Weight Loss and Maintenance In Obese Patients." *Obesity*, 2007; 15 (1): 1464-1472.

Eaton, S. Boyd, M.D., Marjorie Shostak, and Melvin Konner, M.D. PhD. *The Paleo Prescription*. New York: Harper and Row, 1988.

Eaton, SB, and M Konner. "Paleolithic Nutrition: A Consideration of Its Nature and Current Implications." *New England Journal of Medicine*, 1985; 312(5): 283-289.

Fagot-Campagna, A., Burrows, NR, and Williamson, DF. "The Public Health Epidemiology of Type 2 Diabetes in Children and Adolescents: A Case Study of "American Indian Adolescents In the Southwestern United States." *Clinical Chimica Acta*, 1999; 286 (1-2): 81-95.

Fontana, L, and Klein, S. "Aging, Adiposity, and Calorie Restriction." *Journal of the American Medical Association*, 2007 Mar; 297(9): 986-994.

Fontana, L., Klein,S. , and Holloszy, J. "Long-Term, Low-Protein, Low-Calorie Diet and Endurance Exercise Modulates Metabolic Factors Associated With Cancer Risk." *American Journal of Clinical Nutrition*, 2006 Dec; 84(6): 1456-1462.

Forbes.com. 7 December 2006 "The Most Fattening Cocktails." http://www.forbes.com/2006/12/06/fattening-drinks-cocktails-forbeslife-cx_1207cocktails.html.

Ford, ES, Giles, WH, and Dietz, WH. "Prevalence of the Metabolic Syndrome Among US Adults: Findings From the Third National Health and Nutrition Examination Survey." *Journal of the American Medical Association*, 2002 Jan; 287(3): 356-359.

Fritsch, Jane. "95% Regain Lost Weight. Or Do They?" *The New York Times*. 25 May 1999.

Galassi, A, and Reynolds, K. "Metabolic Syndrome and Risk of Cardiovascular Disease: A Meta-Analysis." *The American Journal of Medicine*, 2006;119(10): 812-819.

Gilmore, Gerry J. "Recruit Attrition Falls Across the Services." United States Department of Defense. 13 August 2001, http://www.defenselink.mil/news/newsarticle.aspx?id=44782.

Gorin, A., et al. "Promoting Long-Term Weight Control: Does Dieting Consistency Matter?" *International Journal of Obesity*, 2004; 28: 278-281.

Grodstein, F, et al. "Three-Year Follow-Up of Participants in a Commercial Weight Loss Program: Can You Keep it Off?" *Archives of Internal Medicine*,1996; 156(12): 1302-1306.

Gross, Lee S., et al. "Increased Consumption of Refined Carbohydrates and the Epidemic of Type 2 Diabetes in the United States: An Ecologic Assessment." *American Journal of Clinical Nutrition*, 2004 May; 79(5): 774-779.

"Half Their Size." *People*. 14 Jan. 2008

Harris, JA, and FG Benedict. "A Biometric Study of Basal Metabolism in Man." Proceeding of the National Academy of Sciences, 1918; 4 (12): 370-3.

Heilbronn, L., et al. "Effect of 6-Month Calorie Restriction on Biomarkers of Longevity, Metabolic Adaptation, and Oxidative Stress In Overweight Individuals." *Journal of the American Medical Association*, 2006 Apr; 295(13): 1539-1548.

Henig, RM. "Fat Factors." *New York Times Magazine*. 13 Aug. 2006: 55.

Heshka, S., et al. "Resting Energy Expenditure In the Obese: A Cross-Validation and Comparison of Prediction Equations." *Journal of the American Dietetic Association*, 1993 Sept; 93(9): 1031-1036.

Heymsfield, SB, et al. "Why Do Obese Patients Not Lose More Weight When Treated With Low Calorie Diets?: A Mechanistic Perspective." *American Journal of Clinical Nutrition*, 2007; 8(3): 346-354.

History of Burger King. http://www.entrepreneur.com/franchises/burgerkingcorp/284266-0.html.

History of Flour Enrichment. http://www.gmiflour.com/gmflour/ourheritage.aspx.

History of McDonald's. http://www.globaled.org/curriculum/ffood4.html.

History of Sugar. http://www.sucrose.com

History of Whole Grains. http://www.wholegrainsbureau.ca/about_wg/history_of_wg.html.

IES National Center for Education Statistics. 10 Sept. 2007 http://www.nces.ed.gov.

"In Climbing Mount Everest, Survival Rates Favor the Under 40 Crowd." *The New York Times*. Science Section. 16 May 2007 http://www.nytimes.com/2007/08/21/science/21obclim.html?ref=fitnessandnutrition

References

"Insulin." Wikipedia. http://en.wikipedia.org/wiki/Insulin

Jones, TF, Pavlin BL, La Fleur BJ et al. "Restaurant Inspection Scores and Foodborne Disease." *Emerging Infectious Diseases* (Apr. 2004): http://www.cdc.gov/ncidod/Eid/vol10no4/pdfs/03-0343.pdf.

Katz, David, M.D. MPH. *Looking Good Now Magazine*, interview. June 2006.

Kavanaugh, K., et al. "Trans Fat Diet Induces Abdominal Obesity and Changes in Insulin Sensitivity in Monkeys." *Obesity*, 2007 Jul; 15(7): 1675-1684.

Key, TJ, Schatzkin A, Willett WC, Allen NE, Spencer EA and Travis RC. "Diet, Nutrition, and the Prevention of Cancer." *Public Health Nutrition*, 2004 Feb; 7(1A): 187-200.

King, D, Mainous, A, and Geesey, M. "Turning Back the Clock: Adopting a Healthy Lifestyle in Middle Age." *American Journal of Medicine*, 2007 Jul; 120(7): 598-603.

Klein, S., and Corkey, B., eds. "Mechanism for Metabolic Dysregulation Associated with Obesity." *Obesity*, 2006 Feb; 14:Supplement 1.

Kleinfeld, NR. "Modern Ways to Open India's Doors to Diabetes." *The New York Times*. 13 Sept. 2006.

Klem, M., and Wing, R., et al. "A Descriptive Study of Individuals Successful at Long-Term Weight Maintenance of Substantial Weight Loss." *American Journal of Clinical Nutrition*, 1997; 66: 239-246.

Lazar, MA. "How Obesity Causes Diabetes: Not a Tall Tale." *Science*, 2005 Jan; 307(5708):373-375.

Leibel, R., J. Hirsch, and Et al. "Energy Intake Required to Maintain Body Weight Is Not Affected by Wide Variation in Diet Composition." *American Journal of Clinical Nutrition*, 1992; 55: 350-355.

Leibel, R., M. Rosenbaum, and J.Hirsch. "Changes in Energy Expenditure Resulting From Altered Body Weight." *New England Journal of Medicine*, 1995; 332 (10): 621-628.

Lindeberg, S., Jonsson, T, Granfeldt, Y, Borgstrand,E, Soffman, J,Sjostrom K, Ahren B. "A Palaeolithic Diet Improves Glucose Tolerance More Than a Mediterranean-like Diet In Individuals With Ischaemic Heart Disease." *Diabetologia*, 2007 Jun 22;: 17583796.

Malone, Margaret. "Medications Associated with Weight Gain." *Annals of Pharmacotherapy*, 2005 Dec; 39: 2046-2055.

Mattson, M., R. Cutler, and S. Camandola. "Energy Intake and Amyotrophic Lateral Sclerosis." *NeuroMolecular Medicine*, 2007; 9: 17-20.

Mattson, Mark, PhD. "Gene-Diet Interactions in Brain Aging and Neurodegenerative Disorders." *Annals of Internal Medicine*, 2003; 139: 441-444.

Maynard, LM, et al. "Secular Trends In Desired Weight of Adults." *International Journal of Obesity*, 2006; 30: 1375-1381.

McGuire, MT, Wing, R., and Hill, JO. "The Prevalence of Weight Loss Maintenance Among American Adults." *International Journal of Obesity*, 1999; 23: 1314-1319.

"McDonald's 24/7." *BusinessWeek*. 5 Feb. 2007: 66-72

Mechanism of Sperm Motility. http://www2.oakland.edu/biology/lindemann/SPERM%20FACTS.htm

Role for the Glycemic Index In Preventing Or Treating Diabetes?" *American Journal of Clinical Nutrition*, 2008 Jan; 87(1):1-2 .

Milton, K. "Diet and Primate Evolution." *Scientific American*. 269 (Aug. 1993): 83-93.

Milton, Katherine. "Ferment In the Family Tree." *Integrative and Comparative Biology*, 2004; 44: 304-314.

Mount Everest Facts, http://teacher.scholastic.com/activities/hillary/archive/evefacts.htm.

"Moving to Home Ownership 1994-2002." US Census Bureau. Sept. 2003 http://www.census.gov/prod/2003pubs/h121-03-1.pdf

Neel, JV. "Diabetes Mellitus: A 'Thrifty' Genotype Rendered Detrimental by 'Progress?" *American Journal of Human Genetics*, 1962; 14: 353-362.

Nestle, Marion. "The Soft Sell: How the Food Industry Shapes Our Diets." *Nutrition Action Healthletter*. Sept. 2002.

Nestle, Marion. *What to Eat*. New York: North Point Press, 2006.

O'Dea, Kerin. "Marked Improvement in Carbohydrate and Lipid Metabolism on Diabetic Australian Aborigines After Temporary Reversion to Traditional Lifestyle."*Diabetes*, 1984; 33: 596-603.

O'Keefe, J., and L. Cordain. "Cardiovascular Disease Resulting From a Diet and Lifestyle at Odds With Our Paleolithic Genome: How to Become a 21st-Century Hunter-Gatherer." Mayo Clinic Proceedings, 2004; 79: 101-108.

"Panel Urges FDA Not to Approve Weight-Loss Drug." *The Washington Post*. 14 June 2007: A 08.

Parikh, N, and Et al. "Increasing Trends In Incidence of Overweight and Obesity Over 5 Decades." *The American Journal of Medicine*, 2007; 120: 242-250.

References

Parker-Pope, Tara. "What You Need to Know About Restaurant Dining." *The Wall Street Journal.* 12 Dec. 2006, no. 1 ed.

Pencina, MJ, et al. "Estimated Risks for Developing Obesity in the Framingham Heart Study." *Circulation,* 2006; 113(25):2914-2918.

Phelan, S, et al. "Lessons From Patients Who Have Successfully Maintained Weight Loss." *Obesity Management,* 2005; 1(2): 56-61.

Picard, F., and L. Guarente. "Molecular Links Between Aging and Adipose Tissue." *International Journal of Obesity,* 2005; 29: S36-S39.

Pi-Sunyer, Xavier. "Glycemic Index In Early Type 2 Diabetes." *American Journal of Clinical Nutrition,* 2008; 87: 3-4

Pollan, Michael. *In Defense of Food: An Eater's Manifesto.* New York: Penguin Press, 2008.

Pollan, Michael. Interview on the beef industry, by Terry Gross, Radio WHYY. 3 Apr. 2002.

Pollan, Michael. *The Omnivore's Dilemma.* New York: Penguin Books, 2006.

"Practice Tips: How to Intervene With Overweight and Obese Patients." *The American Journal of Medicine* / Editorial, 2005; 118: 936-938.

Ramachandran, V., et al. "Estimated Risks for Developing Obesity in the Framingham Heart Study." *Annals of Internal Medicine,* 2005; 143: 473-480.

Roberts, W. "Salt and Blood Pressure." Proceedings of Baylor University Medical Center, 2001 Jul; 14(3): 314-322.

Rolls, BJ. "Experimental Analyses of the Effects of Variety In a Meal on Human Feeding." *American Journal of Clinical Nutrition,* 1985; 42: 932-939.

Roth, J. "The Obesity Pandemic: Where Have We Been and Where Are We Going?" *Obesity Research,* 2004 Nov; 12: Supplement

Ryan, A., Nicklas, B., and Berman, D. "Aerobic Exercise Is Necessary To Improve Glucose Utilization With Moderate Weight Loss In Women." *Obesity,* 2006 Jun;,14 (6):1064-1072.

Sahyoun, N., Anderson, A., et al. "Dietary Glycemic Index and Glycemic Load and the Risk of Type 2 Diabetes In Older Adults." *American Journal of Clinical Nutrition,* 2008; 87: 126-131.

Schlosser, Eric. *Fast Food Nation.* New York: Perennial, 2002.

Schwartz, Barry. *The Paradox of Choice.* New York: Harper Collins, 2004.

Shelmet, J., Reichard G., et al. "Ethanol Causes Acute Inhibition of Carbohydrate, Fat and Protein Oxidation and Insulin Resistance." *Journal of Clinical Investigation,* 1988; 81: 1137-1145.

Siler, S.Q., Neese, R.A., and Hellerstein, M.K. "De Novo Lipogenesis, Lipid Kinetics, and Whole-Body Lipid Balances in Humans After Acute Alcohol Consumption." *American Journal of Clinical Nutrition*, 1999;70: 928-936.

Silva, M, et al. "Adult Obesity and Number of Years Lived With and Without Cardiovascular Disease." *Obesity*, 2006 July; 14(7):164-1273.

Sonnenberg, L.,Pencina, M., et al. "Dietary Patterns and the Metabolic Syndrome in Obese and Non-Obese Framingham Women." *Obesity Research*, 2005;13:153-162.

Stevens, J., et al. "The Definition of Weight Maintenance." *International Journal of Obesity*, 2006; 30: 391-399.

Storey, M, and French, S. "Food Advertising and Marketing Directed at Children and Adolescents in the US." *International Journal of Behavioral Nutrition and Physical Activity*, 2004; 1 (3).

Super Bowl Ads, 4 February 2008 http://money.cnn.com/2008/02/04/news/companies/superbowl_ads/index.htm.

Taubes, Gary. *Good Calories, Bad Calories*. New York: Alfred A. Knopf, 2007.

"The IDF Consensus Worldwide Definition of the Metabolic Syndrome." International Diabetes Federation. 22 Sept. 2007 http://www.idf.org/webdata/docs/MetS_def_update2006.pdf

"The State of Physical Activity and Nutrition Education in Illinois," http://www.acfn.org/resources/IL.

"Time to Pinch Off the Salt." *American Medical News*. 2008; 51 (2).

"Trans Fats: The Story Behind the Label." Harvard School of Public Health. http://www.hsph.harvard.edu/review/rvw_spring06/rvwspr06_transfats.html.

"Unhappy Meals." *New York Times Magazine* / Cover Article. 28 Jan. 2007.

Van Dale, D., Saris,WHM, and Ten Hoor, F. "Weight Maintenance and Resting Metabolic Rate 18-40 Months After a Diet-Exercise Treatment." *International Journal of Obesity*, 1990;14: 347-359.

Varady, K., and Hellerstein, M. "Alternate-Day Fasting and Chronic Disease Prevention: A Review of Human and Animal Trials." *American Journal of Clinical Nutrition*, 2007; 86: 7-13.

Vogels, N., and Westerterp-Plantenga, MS. "Categorical Strategies Based On Subject Characteristics of Dietary Restraint and Physical Activity For Weight Maintenance." *International Journal of Obesity*, 2005; 29: 849-857.

References

Walker, A., Walker, B., and Adam, F. "Nutrition, Diet, Physical Activity, Smoking and Longevity: From Primitive Hunter-Gatherer to Present Passive Consumer--How Far Can We Go?" *Nutrition*, 2003;19: 169-173.

Wansink, B., Painter, J., and North, J. "Bottomless Bowls: Why Visual Cues of Portion Size May Influence Intake." *Obesity Research*, 2005 Jan; 13: 93-100.

Wansink, Brian. Mindless Eating. New York: Bantam Books, 2006.

Warnberg, J., et al. "Inflammatory Proteins Are Related To Total and Abdominal Adiposity In a Healthy Adolescent Population: The AVENA study." *American Journal of Clinical Nutrition*, 2006; 84: 505-512.

Weight Maintenance Statistics. National Weight Control Registry. http://www.nwcr.ws/Research/default.htm.

"Weight Management Using a Meal Replacement Strategy: Meta and Pooling Analysis From Six Studies." *Int J Obes Relat Metab Disord*, 2003; 27: 537-549.

Weil, Andrew, M.D. *Eating Well for Optimum Health*. New York: Alfred A. Knopf, 2000.

Weindruch, R., and Sohal,RS. "Caloric Intake and Aging." *New England Journal of Medicine*, 1997; 337: 986-994.

Wendy's Information , http:/www.Wendys.com

Westerterp, K., Smeets, A., et al. "The Canadian Trial of Carbohydrates in Diabetes, a 1-Y Controlled Trial of Low-Glycemic-Index Dietary Carbohydrate In Type 2 Diabetes: "No Effect On Glycated Hemoglobin But Reduction in C-Reactive Protein." *American Journal of Clinical Nutrition*, 2008; 87(1):114-125.

Westerterp-Plantenga, M. "Successful Long-Term Weight Maintenance: A 2-Year Follow-Up." *Obesity*, 2007 May; 15 (5): 1258-1266.

Westman, E., R. Feinman, and Et al. "Low-Carbohydrate Nutrition and Metabolism." *American Journal of Clinical Nutrition*, 2007;86: 276-284.

Willett, WC, Stampfer, M., et al. "Intake of Trans Fatty Acids and Risk of Coronary Heart Disease Among Women." *Lancet*, 1993; 341: 581-585.

Willett. Walter. *Eat, Drink and Be Healthy*. New York: Free Press, 2001.

Wing, R, and Hill, J. "Successful Weight Loss Maintenance." *Annual Review Nutrition*, 2001; 21: 323-341.

Wing, R., and Jeffery, R. "Food Provision As a Strategy to Promote Weight Loss." Obesity Research Supplement, 2001 Nov; 4: 271S-275S.

Wyatt, H., et al. "Lessons from Patients Who Have Successfully Maintained Weight Loss." *Obesity Management*, 2005; 1(2): 56-61.

Yan, Lijing L., et al. "Midlife Body Mass Index and Hospitalization and Mortality in Older Age." *Journal of the American Medical Association*, 2006; 295: 90-198.

Index

Index

Index